How to be Your Own Health Visitor

The Complete Guide to Breast or Bottle Feeding, Weaning, Sleeping, Immunisation, Growth and Development, Behavioural Issues and much more.

Ann Guindi

© 2014 Ann Guindi

No part of this publication may be reproduced or transmitted in any form by any means, electronic or mechanical, including photocopy, recording, or information storage and retrieval methods now known, or to be invented, without the written permission of Ann Guindi, except by a reviewer who wishes to quote brief passages in connection with a review written for inclusion in an educational publication or radio or TV broadcast.

Contact information:
ann@parentingpeace.co.uk
www.parentingpeace.co.uk

Foreword

Ann Guindi is the founder of *Parenting Peace,* an organisation that has been set up in order to help new parents in their most important life role – parenting. We will give you education, mentoring and coaching through all your challenges. We all know that your babies/children do not come with an instruction manual and this can be quite a daunting experience to be completely responsible for your most precious possession. Don't worry, we are here to help ease your concerns and to make your parenting experience as enjoyable and stress free as possible.

Our vision is to bring peace to every parent and enable you to be confident and knowledgeable in the choices you make for your baby.

Ann has worked with children for the past 30yrs, starting out as a sick children's nurse. Ann has been a health visitor for over 20yrs and is passionate about the promotion of health and the prevention of ill health.

She is now putting all her knowledge, skills and experience into her first book, in order to help you, the parent, to be the parent that you want to be.

Ann set up *Parenting* Peace because she is passionate about Parenting and knows, as a Mother of four children how challenging and rewarding it can be.

There are many books out there on parenting and "how to" do it; this, is not one of those books. In her roles parent educator, mentor and coach, Ann believes you will find your own style that is unique to you and your baby. The focus of this book is to provide you with the knowledge and education so you can make an informed decision as to how you want to raise your child.

Acknowledgements

To my family, my darling husband Chris who encourages me in everything I do and every endeavour I take on. Thank you for believing in me and being my greatest fan. To my four wonderful children; Ben, Joe, Ollie and Sophie; you have taught me so much over the last twenty years as your mother. I apologise for the times that I was not a 'good enough' mother.

To all the mother's that I have had the pleasure to work with over the past twenty years. It has been an honour to serve and learn from you all as your health visitor. You have allowed me into your home and your lives and it has been a pleasure to help you through the good times and the not so good times.

For all of the colleagues that I have worked alongside over the last 30 years and those who have supported me in my career and journey into being a better health visitor.

A big thank you to all those who read my book for content; Helen, Ramona, Gina and a special thank you to my good friend and colleague Louise for all the valuable feedback given to me.

Table of Contents

Introduction 1

   Chapter One – Welcome to Parenthood 3

      Why did I Write this Book? 3

      Who am I and What Right do I have to Write this book? 3

      What is a Health Visitor? 4

      So What Specifically do They do? 5

      What to Expect From Your Health Visitor 5

      The Healthy Child Programme (HCP) 7

      The Antenatal Contact Visit 7

      Genogram/Family Tree 8

      Family Needs Assessment 11

      Parenting Capacity 11

      Health Behaviour 12

      Physical and Mental Health Issues 12

      Family and Environmental Factors 12

      Child's Developmental Needs 13

      My Personal Story 17

      Early Hospital Interventions 18

      Hearing Screening 18

      Other Screening and Surveillance 18

      The Midwife Input 19

      Health Visitor Input - New Birth Visit (7-14 day) 21

      Mother 22

      Follow-up Visit 22

- Developmental Assessments 23
- 6-8 week developmental check 23
- 8-12Mt Developmental Check 25
- 2-2.5yr Developmental Check 26
- Targeted 3.5yr check 26
- Conclusion 26

Chapter Two - How to be Your own Health Visitor 28

Background 29

Post Birth Check (within 72 hrs of birth) 29

New birth Visit 31
- Birth Details and Newborn Examination 33
- Physical Check of Baby 33
- Head 34
- Eyes 35
- Jaundice 35
- Nose 37
- Mouth 38
- Tongue-Tie 39
- Skin 40
- Nappy area 40
- Circumcision 41

Prevention of Cot Death/Sudden Infant Death Syndrome (SIDS) 44
- What can I do to help prevent SIDS? 44
- Follow the advice below to help prevent SIDS: 44

Chapter Three - Immunisations 46
- Childhood Immunisation Programme 46

Immunisations 46

What is BCG Vaccine? 47

What is TB? 47

How is it transferred? 47

Symptoms 47

How is my Baby Immunised? 48

Side Effects 48

What is Diphtheria? 50

What is Tetanus? 50

What is Pertussis (Whooping Cough)? 51

What is Polio? 51

What is Hib? 51

What is Pneumococcal Vaccine? 52

What is Meningococcal C? 52

MMR Vaccine (Measles, Mumps and Rubella) 52

What is Measles? 52

What is Mumps? 53

What is Rubella? 53

Advice to Parents after Your Child Has Been Immunised 54

General Reactions 54

Persistent Crying or Screaming 54

Prolonged Severe Fever 54

Convulsions or Fits 55

Local Reactions 55

Rashes 56

Chapter Four – Maternal Health and Well Being 58

General Advice Given to Parent at New Birth Visit 58

Registration of Birth and with GP 58

Benefits 61

Physical Assessment of Mother 62

Personal Story 62

Breast care 65

Common Problems 66

Initiating Breastfeeding/Skin-to-Skin Contact/Rooming-in 67

Storing Breast Milk 71

Avoid Use of Dummies 71

Avoid Supplementary Feeding 72

Post-Natal Check and Exercises 73

Contraception 74

Cervical Screening 75

Maternal Mood Assessment 76

EDINBURGH POSTNATAL DEPRESSION SCALE (EPDS) 78

EDINBURGH POSTNATAL DEPRESSION SCALE SCORE SHEET 81

Chapter Five - Bottle Feeding 87

How to Recognise Signs of When Your Baby Wants to Feed 87

Bottle Feeding 87

Addition of Nutrients to Formula 89

Types of Milk 89

Standard Infant Formula 90

Vitamin D Supplements 91

Signs and Symptoms of Low Levels 91

Case Study 92

Follow-on Formula 92

Cow's Milk.. 93

Goat's and Sheep's milk 94

Soya Infant Formulas... 95

Cow's Milk Protein Allergy (CMPA) 96

Personal Story 96

Pre-term Babies 99

How do I Encourage my Baby to Feed Correctly From a Bottle? .. 99

Bottles and Teats.. 100

Wind 101

Causes of Wind in Breast-Fed Babies 101

Causes of Wind in Bottle-Fed Babies.. 102

How Often Should I Feed my Baby?... 102

Colic.. 103

Management... 103

Drug Treatment... 104

Chapter Six- Health Education and Promotion................................. 105

Clinic Visits 105

Percentile/Growth Charts.. 105

How to Interpret the Graph 106

Growth Charts Taken from Parent-Held Record/Red book........ 107

Top 10 Questions Asked of Health Visitors 109

Other Minor Problems 121

What is Constipation? 121

Breastfed Babies 122

Bottle-Fed Babies 122

- Older Children 123
- What is Diarrhoea? 124
- Dehydration 125
- Prevention and Treatment of Dehydration 125
- Older Children 126

Chapter Seven – You and Your Baby's First Year 127

- Follow up Home Visit by Health Visitor (6-8 weeks) 128
  - Baby 128
  - Mother 128
- First Developmental Check 6-8 weeks 129
- Why Attend this Developmental Check? 130
- Case Study 131
- 3-4 month Home Visit (Not All Families Will be Offered This Visit) 132
  - Weaning onto Solids 132
  - Cutting Down on Milk Feeds 133
  - Foods to Avoid 135
  - Gag Reflux 135
  - Dental Hygiene 136
  - Drinks 136
  - Returning to Work 137
  - Childcare 137
  - Family 138
  - Child-minder 138
  - Nursery 138
  - Nanny 139
  - Au-Pairs 139

  Share Between You and Your Partner 140

Chapter Eight- Sleep and Behaviour 141

  Why is Sleep so Important? 141

  The Impact of Sleep Deprivation on Children 141

  The Impact of Sleep Deprivation on Parents 142

  What is a Sleep Problem? 142

  Advantages of a Good Sleep Pattern 143

  How to Teach Your Child to Sleep 143

  Method One - Gradual Retreat 145

  Method Two –Controlled Crying 146

  Personal Story 147

  Older Child Who Repeatedly Gets Out of Bed 148

  Nightmares 148

  Night Terrors 149

 Behaviour Issues 150

  Temper Tantrums 150

 Sibling Rivalry 152

  Aggressive Behaviour 154

  Prevention 154

  Help Them Learn Empathy 155

  Redirection or Distraction 156

  Positive Behaviour 157

Chapter Nine - Development 159

 Baby/Child Assessments/Developmental Checks 159

 Emotional/Intellectual Development 159

 7-11 Month Developmental Check 163

2 Year Developmental Check 169
    Personal story 172
Bonus Chapter One 177
Chapter Ten - The Theory and Practice of Learning and Development
.... 177
    Neuroscience 177
Psychological Development 177
    Behaviourism 178
    Social Learning Theory 178
    Constructivism 179
Social Constructivism 180
    Old Thinking: 181
    New Thinking 182
How Can You Stimulate Your Baby in the Five Areas of Development?
.... 183
    Activities for Babies 8-12 Months Old 183
    Communication 183
    Fine Motor 183
    Gross Motor 184
    Problem Solving 185
    Personal Social 186
Activities for Children 24-30 Months old 186
    Communication 186
    Fine Motor 187
    Gross Motor 187
    Problem Solving 188
    Personal Social 189

Summary	190
Bonus Chapter Two	191
Chapter Eleven - The Importance of Parenting	191
Why did you Become a Parent?	191
What is a Parent?	191
Why is Parenting Important?	192
The Importance of Parenting in the Early Years	193
What Type of Parent Are You?	193
1. Authoritarian	193
2. Permissive Parenting	194
3. Democratic Parenting	195
Attachment Theory	196
Secure Attachment	197
Insecure Attachment	197
The Importance of Knowing Your Baby's Personality	198
Temperament	199
To Conclude	209
Bibliography	211
About the Author	213

Introduction

It is a 150 years since the first health visitor (HV) provided support to new families in the UK. I have been very fortunate to work as a HV for a quarter of a century. I have seen many changes in the role in that time. Sadly, HV numbers have been steadily declining in the last 10 years which has had a negative impact on maternal health and wellbeing, as the service has been compromised for some years now. In an effort to address this, in 2011 the Government responded by introducing the 'Health Visitor Implementation Plan 2011-2015' (for more information visit www.dh.gov.uk/implementationplan) by placing funding into recruiting an extra 4,200 HVs by 2015. By that time, 60-70% of the profession will have been trained in the last three years. That will mean a huge loss of knowledge and expertise in those experienced HVs retiring, hence me writing this book.

The purpose of this book is to give all new and not so new parents, the knowledge, skills and experience that I have gained over the last 30yrs in working with both sick and well children. It is my hope that by reading this book it may enable you, the reader, to absorb some of that knowledge so you can make informed decisions for your child. I feel knowledge is power. My focus will be on the role of the HV in your child's early years.

As a parent to four children I know how difficult it was at times for me. I thought I would sail through parenting; after all, I was a professional health visitor when I had my first baby. But I still felt overwhelmed at times, especially in the early days of parenthood. I also made lots of mistakes along the way. I want to give you my perspective both as a professional and a mother. There are many books on parenting out there in the market but no other book will give you an insider's professional viewpoint, coupled with the reality of being a parent.

Introduction

I hope you will enjoy the book and the experience of being a parent; after all there is no better job in the world.

Chapter One – Welcome to Parenthood

Why did I write this book?

I wrote this book because babies do not come with an instruction manual. One of the biggest myths about parenting is that it comes naturally and it may well do to some of you lucky parents. But I wrote this book for all those parents who, like me, found it hard work and learned on the job by making mistakes. I thought I knew quite a lot having learned all the theory but let me tell you it soon went out the window when my emotions were involved. I seemed to lose all logic once I became a parent. But despite my highly emotional state I managed to muddle through and yes, my training did give me the knowledge, and on a good day the confidence to get through the challenging times.

Who am I and what right do I have to write this book?

I started my nurse training in 1982 having qualified as a Sick Children's Nurse. I worked in hospitals for 8 years looking after many hundreds of sick children and supporting their parents. However, I became concerned about how many children came into hospital that should never have ended up there, if only their parents could have received the correct support and education to prevent an admission. So in 1990 I trained as a health visitor (HV) to help parents in the promotion of health and the prevention of ill health.

I loved my job so much I remained active as a HV for over 20 years and have advised many thousands of mothers in that time. But most importantly I am a mother to my own four children. My eldest son,

Chapter One: Welcome to Parenthood

Ben, my eldest, is now 19 years old and at university. My second son, Joe, is preparing for A levels. My third eldest son, Ollie, is 14 years old and a typical teenager, whilst my only daughter, Sophie, is 10 years old and in her last year at primary school. However, I still remember clearly the day each one of them was born and also remember the trials and challenges I faced as a new mother, all too well. I have been where you have been and went through all the excitement, worry and all the other many emotions of being a parent.

When I had my first baby I already had over a decade of working with both sick children in hospital and well children, as I had been working as a HV for 4 years before giving birth to Ben. I thought that I had all the knowledge, skills and experience that I needed to become a great mother. But if I am honest it was the biggest shock of my life. I will explain more on that later.

What is a Health Visitor?

Well, if you are a first time mum you will probably never even have heard of a Health Visitor (HV) but are probably curious or else you would not be reading this book. A HV is a unique role and they are specific to UK. There are similar roles in other countries but of a different name; for example in Ireland they would be known as the Public Health Nurse. HVs primarily work with families to support parents of children under five years old. They are qualified nurses and pre 2011 would have had at least two years of experience in their chosen field. In addition, most would have had a further qualification in midwifery or sick children nursing. As I mentioned earlier, there is currently a shortage of HVs nationally and the Government is trying to address this by introducing the 'Implementation Plan' and recruiting additional HVs. As a result, nurses will now have direct entry into health visiting following qualification as a nurse. However, all will have to undergo specialist training before qualifying to work with you and your baby.

So what specifically do they do?

The role of the HV is to advise, guide and support you, the parent, through the first five years of parenting. They do this by offering health education and promotion through a combination of home visits and clinic attendance. They carry out developmental surveillance screening on your baby throughout various stages of your baby's development. However, I know that that this service will vary with each individual HV and where you live. I cannot reiterate enough that the service will vary throughout the UK depending on what the commissioners in your area buy into.

A Netmums survey which asked more than 6,000 mothers on their views of HVs in 2008 revealed that women were grateful for the support they received but that it was not always enough, and that access to HVs across the UK was patchy.

What to expect from your Health Visitor

Sadly, as mentioned previously, this will vary depending on the individual HV and where you live. Although the role is similar the amount of contact will be governed by availability of staff and the commissioners in that specific area. Many HVs will be attached to a health centre and others are attached to children centres. Some are attached to a GP Practice and others work a specific geographical area.

Chapter One: Welcome to Parenthood

Many HVs now work in corporate caseloads. This means that the work load is shared amongst the team. This could mean that you may not see the same HV on a regular or continuous basis but may see one of her colleagues. Many Healthcare Trusts are now trying to ensure that there is more continuity after your baby is born in that you see the same HV at least twice or three times to build a relationship, but there is no guarantee due to staff pressures. You will always be seen for the first visit by a qualified HV in order to make a full assessment of your families health needs but then the care may be handed over to a member of the skill mix team.

What does skill mix mean? Skill mix is a mixed ability team where each individual working within the team will have different qualifications and skills. The HV will head the team and take accountability for decisions made in the delivery of each family's care. The HV is then supported by Community Staff Nurses (CSN) who are qualified midwives or nurses (general, mental health or paediatric) who will be competent in working with the sick, as they mainly will have come from working in the acute sector i.e. hospitals. But, they will have carried out induction training to work within the community. There will also be nursery nurses (NN) who are qualified in child development and may have come from an education setting i.e. nursery/schools and they will work alongside the HV carrying out home visits and developmental checks. Many Trusts will operate in this way; however, there will be variations. I would recommend asking your HV how their particular service operates within your area.

The Department of Health (DOH) states:

"Pregnancy and the first years of life are one of most important stages in the life cycle. This is when the foundations of future health and wellbeing are being laid down, and it's a time when parents are particularly receptive to learning and making changes. There is good evidence that outcomes for both children and adults are strongly influenced by the factors that operate during pregnancy and the first years of life".

The Healthy Child Programme (HCP)

The Healthy Child Programme (HCP) begins in early pregnancy and ends at adulthood. For more information visit www.dh.gov.uk/healthychildprogramme .

The core requirements of the HCP are;

- Early identification of need and risk
- Health and development reviews
- Screening

The first contact will be in pregnancy by the midwife and should be carried out by 10 weeks of pregnancy. There will be ten visits to your midwife in total (recommended and for first baby only). Antenatal screening for fetal conditions will be carried out according to NICE guidelines. I will not be covering the role of the midwife in this book as I am not qualified to do so.

The Antenatal Contact Visit

This visit will be the first point of contact with your HV and the purpose is to introduce the service and taking time getting to know one another. It will take about an hour to an hour and a half to complete this initial visit.

Antenatal visits will only be offered to first time mothers and those who are deemed to be more vulnerable. By vulnerable I mean those who may have difficulties after the baby is born due to some underlying health needs or other concerns around their capacity to

Chapter One: Welcome to Parenthood

cope as a parent. This is very subjective and based on sparse information received from the midwife in the antenatal notification. When the antenatal assessment visit is carried out by the HV it will be more objective having spent time with the parents-to-be in the home environment.

The exact timing of the antenatal contact will vary again from area to area but most likely to be in the last trimester mainly due to most mothers being at work and unavailable. During this visit the HV will be getting to know you and building a relationship with you. They will subtlety be observing the home environment and making an assessment about the cleanliness of the home but not in an obvious way. Relax, don't worry, they will not be carrying out a home inspection and going from room to room giving you marks out of ten! I know many mothers that have been spent hours deep cleaning their home before the HV arrived to make a good impression. HVs just want to ensure that the house is generally tidy and safe for a baby to be living in without any risk to health.

Genogram/Family Tree

In some areas a genogram or family tree will form part of the HVs assessment, but it is not common practice. Some people find this quite invasive and you may feel that it is not relevant. But this will give the HV an overall picture of your family make up and any health needs that are in your family or health needs that may be passed down to your baby like asthma, eczema and diabetes, for example. But it also gives a good understanding of who is around to support you after the baby is born and research suggests that mothers who have better support are less likely to become depressed after birth. I know many single mothers and mothers who have no family living near them, to be well supported by friends and neighbours and this is equally important. If

Chapter One: Welcome to Parenthood

there is no support it is of course much harder for the parents, especially when the father goes back to work.

A typical genogram should include three generations.

What do the shapes represent?

A square = Male

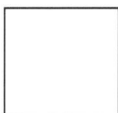

A circle = Female

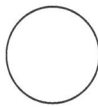

Triangle = Unknown sex

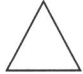

✚ = Death

X = Miscarriage/Termination

Unions

Continuous line = current or enduring relationship

Dotted line = Transitory relationship

Severed/crossed out line = separation/broken relationship

See example overleaf:

(Twins are normally illustrated slightly differently but I have done it my way on purpose for clearer illustration).

Chapter One: Welcome to Parenthood

Example:

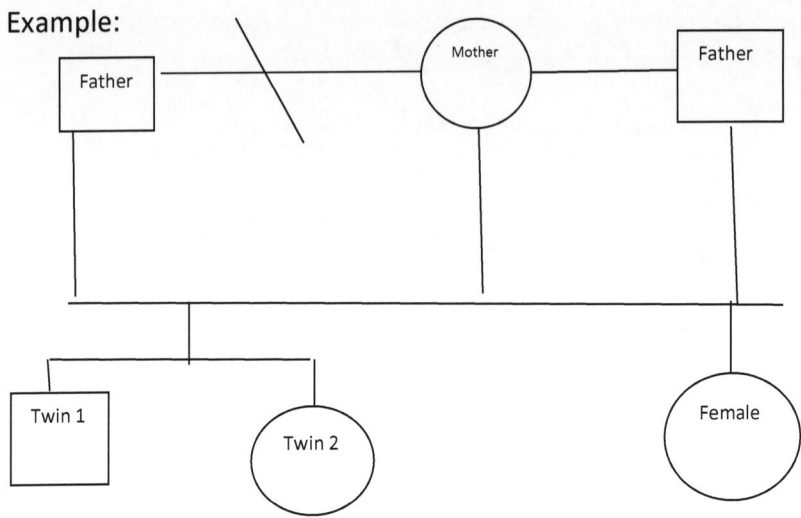

So if we look at the example given above, we can see that the mother has had a previous relationship which resulted in a twin pregnancy. The mother is no longer with her ex-partner (crossed out line) but both the children are living with her and her new partner. In this situation it is important to ascertain whether the ex-partner has access to his children and when this occurs. It is also important for the HV to find out the reason behind the breakdown of the relationship, as it may impact on the family.

For example, if the previous partner was violent and the mother left for her own safety and the safety of her children, this may be a concern. It is important that the children are safe; so the HV may ask more questions about the access visits. For example, are they supervised, or if visits are with a family member or in a contact centre. If with a family member then the risk is elevated as there is no guarantee that the supervision is maintained. There may at times be other agencies involved with your family to offer you support like social services or a family support worker. The HV will ask you about the contact details of these people in social services or sure start children's centres as they may want to speak with them to know more about meeting your family's needs.

It is important to stress that HVs are NOT social workers but they will work closely with social workers. Every professional has a duty to protect your children and prevent any risk of harm.

Family Needs Assessment

HVs will want to know about your general health and if you are leading a healthy lifestyle. Again, some topics you may find a little intrusive as they go into deeper personal issues like smoking, drinking, drug-taking and may even ask about any history of domestic violence if it is safe to do so. This will NEVER be asked in front of a partner/husband. These are important areas to explore as they will have an impact on both your health and that of your baby's. They are basically making an assessment of your health needs. But usual topics will include:

Parenting Capacity

- Maternal age
- Maternal health
- Previous pregnancies/ birth experience/SIDS-Sudden Infant Death Syndrome(cot death)
- Current pregnancy – planned/unplanned.
- Booked before 24 weeks of pregnancy
- Attendance at antenatal/parent craft classes
- Birth plan – Whether you want a natural birth or intervention

Chapter One: Welcome to Parenthood

Health Behaviour

- Nutrition and diet
- Exercise
- Smoking, drinking, drug-taking
- Sexual Health/Cervical smear

Physical and Mental Health Issues

- General health status – Asthma, diabetes etc.
- Learning difficulties
- Emotional/psychological health status – Anxiety/depression/panic attacks, bi-polar disorder etc.
- Parent-child interaction

Family and Environmental Factors

- Family health and wellbeing – relevant physical/mental health issues
- Income/benefits/employment/residency status (if not resident there will be no access to public funding)
- Domestic Violence
- Parents experience of being parented
- Housing conditions
- Language/cultural issues
- Current involvement with other organisations/resources

Chapter One: Welcome to Parenthood

Child's Developmental Needs

- Attendance for antenatal screening
- Any potential problems with baby's weight
- Intention to breast/bottle feed
- Attendance at antenatal/parent-craft classes

If you have not attended any antenatal/parent-craft classes I would strongly recommend to take advantage of the free classes run by NHS midwives. They will give you a basic run through of the stages of labour and delivery. They also normally offer you a tour around the delivery suite of your nominated hospital; this will help you when you are in labour - if you are familiar with the environment you are likely to feel less vulnerable. I did this with my first baby even though I was planning a home birth (which did not happen due to complications during labour). I was very glad that I had done this tour as it gave me some reassurance and some control over the situation. The National Childbirth Trust (NCT) also offers some classes but there is a fee involved.

It is important to know that the NCT classes are facilitative and facilitators are not trained midwives. However, all the facilitators will be mothers who have experiential knowledge or that was my personal experience and to my knowledge still is the case today.

However, they offer an excellent service that is sadly not being covered by the NHS. Again the focus is on birth and breathing to help you in labour along with a strong focus on breastfeeding. I really enjoyed my NCT classes as I met up with other parents which provided the social support that is equally important after having a baby. But there was no mention of bottle feeding which was fine for me as I wanted to breastfeed, however, not all women who attend these classes may be successful in their breastfeeding and I feel this may be a disadvantage

Chapter One: Welcome to Parenthood

and a potential risk. As a health visitor I have seen many women who desperately wanted to breastfeed but ended up bottle feeding. These mothers had little knowledge on how to prepare feeds correctly or about sterilisation options and techniques available to them. It also exacerbated their feelings of isolation and failure.

My personal opinion was that this could possibly have been an issue for those parents who wanted to bottle feed; they may have felt a little bit of pressure or a sense of not belonging. I am a firm advocate of breastfeeding but I also will advise and support parents who choose to bottle feed for whatever reason. I feel that there is sometimes too much pressure to be the 'perfect' mother and this can cause much upset when breastfeeding is not achieved. I believe it can cause much harm emotionally. It is perfectly OK to bottle feed. However, I know many of my colleagues may disagree with me and that is fine, we are all entitled to our opinions. I will NEVER make judgements on your choice of feeding.

Following an initial assessment your family will be placed in one of three HV caseloads:

Universal/Core services- receive the services laid down in the Healthy Child Programme and outlined below. For the purposes of this book I will only be talking about families who fall into this caseload.

Universal Plus/Vulnerable families – these families will receive all the core services and additional support as agreed between the family and their HV.

Families that may fall into this category could include any or all of the following:

- Mental health issues
- Domestic violence (DV)

Chapter One: Welcome to Parenthood

- Drug or alcohol problems
- Post natal depression
- Teenage/unsupported mother
- Significant housing issues
- Significant financial issues
- Parenting issues
- Children with special/additional needs

It is important to stress that not all parents who have any of these issues will be deemed as vulnerable as I know some teenage mums that would put any older mother to shame. I also know many women with mental health issues that are stable and wonderful mothers. This is a guide only, if the drug and alcohol issues are in the past then that is different. On the other hand, if the perpetrator of DV is still in the house then the mother and children can be at risk of harm.

Safeguarding/Child Protection families- these families again will receive all the core services but the children will be on a child protection plan or a child in need (CIN) plan. This means that the local authority has deemed the family to be at risk of significant harm and there will be a child protection (CP) plan in place to protect the children from any likely or further abuse (physical, emotional, sexual or neglect). Usually the HV would visit monthly along with a social worker who will visit more frequently to monitor the children and keep them safe.

The second two categories are where HVs spend most of their time, hence the need for introducing skill mix to the health visiting service. Most core services can be and are undertaken by the support team. When I first came into health visiting over 20 years ago there were no skill mix/corporate (shared) caseloads. Instead all HVs had their own caseloads and visited their families from birth right up until school age.

Chapter One: Welcome to Parenthood

This was very rewarding for both the HV and the family as we were able to build a long and lasting relationship of trust. Sadly this does not happen any longer. You will be lucky to see the same HV once or twice during your baby's first year. If you do want continuity it is best to go to the same clinic to have your baby weighed, whether it be to your GP or local community clinic. But again there is no guarantee that it will be the same HV each week. If you are lucky enough to be offered post natal support groups in your area then I would suggest you take full advantage of them as they are few and far between. They will be delivered by the nursery nurses and staff nurses. The reason for this is, as previously mentioned, that nursery nurses are ideally placed to deliver this health education and promotion. However, when I first started out as a HV it was the HVs who delivered all the health education classes. Sadly due to declining numbers in the profession and the demands on HVs to safeguard children this part of their role has become extinct.

However, I must stress that the staff nurses and nursery nurses do a fantastic job and have been trained to deliver these courses. I really loved my job when I was delivering health education and promotion classes, this is why I became a health visitor. I believe that in running these valuable courses, giving health education advice and guidance cuts down on anxiety and depression and prevents attendance at many busy A&E departments. In many areas these classes are not being offered at all due to lack of resources. As a result these classes are now being taken over by other private organisations i.e. NCT or the Pre-school Learning Alliance.

On a personal level, as a mother I found having a baby was the most life changing experience that I have gone through to date. I don't think anything can prepare you for how your life will change. Becoming a parent is one of the best things that has ever happened to me and my life is happy and fulfilled just by having a family to share life with. I was lucky enough to fall completely and utterly in love with my babies when they were born, despite my first labour being a fairly negative experience. However, I know this is not the case for every mother. (Please see next section on post natal depression assessment).

My Personal Story

When I was pregnant with my first baby I was hoping to have a home birth. I had attended all the classes that were available including both hospital and the local NCT group. I was well prepared, or so I thought, for my planned water birth. When my waters broke at home at 5.30am I thought I would go into labour and my baby would be born later that day. But I didn't go into labour straight away, in fact I didn't have any labour pains at all until the evening. I laboured all night without any sleep thinking my baby would be here by morning. The following morning the midwife came and she said I had to go to hospital as it was policy after 24 hrs and it could be a risk to the baby. I was so upset I didn't want to go but reluctantly went. It was then that I felt I'd lost control of my planned natural birth. I was induced and felt pinned to my bed with a drip in one hand and the monitor over my abdomen to trace the baby's heartbeat. When I finally reached full dilation I was exhausted and despite 2 hours of pushing, I was unable to deliver my baby. I ended up with a medical birth - a ventouse (vacuum) extraction after a long hard 36 hr labour. I had lots of stitches and very painful haemorrhoids (piles). I was too shattered to even contemplate breastfeeding.

I tell you this story not to scare you but to advise you that sometimes things don't go to plan. Seeing your HV before birth really helps to build a relationship, which then enables you to feel supported following a difficult birth. But more importantly being prepared for every eventuality is so important.

Early Hospital Interventions

Once your baby is born it is important that they undergo many screening tests to ensure their health and well-being. Your baby will also be offered a vitamin K injection to prevent bleeding in the newborn baby occurring. Most babies will receive this as an injection and you as parents should be asked for consent. Sometimes parents choose to have this by an oral route but your baby will need three doses to be fully protected.

Hearing Screening

Your baby should also have their hearing assessment carried out in the hospital before discharge (sometimes done at home after discharge). This is a painless procedure where a probe is placed into each ear to test for any hearing deficit. There may be times when this procedure is not done in the hospital. For instance, if you choose to return home within hours of the birth or if you deliver at the weekend you will not have the opportunity of getting this procedure completed. However, you will need to have this completed in the community and you should be given an appointment or information on who to contact before discharge.

Other Screening and Surveillance

Chapter One: Welcome to Parenthood

Before your baby even leaves the hospital she/he will have a number of procedures completed. This will include a newborn baby check (I will cover this in detail in the next chapter) and in most cases a neonatal hearing screening test as mentioned above.

The Midwife Input

The midwife should come and see you and your baby at home once you are discharged from hospital. Unfortunately, there is also a shortage of trained midwives and you will probably only be seen once at home. Many midwives are now asking new mothers to come to the hospital or community setting to be seen. At the home visit the midwife will take blood from your baby's heel to test for any underlying blood disorders. This should be completed between day 5-8 after birth. This screening test should be carried out by the midwife at home, if it isn't you need to contact your midwife before you are discharged from her care.

This is an important screening test and includes detection of the following disorders:

- Phenylketonuria (P.K.U)
- Cystic Fibrosis
- Hypothyroidism
- Sickle cell anaemia/Thallasceamia
- MCADD (Medium-chain acyl-CoA dehydronase deficiency

If there are any concerns with you or your baby your midwife will continue to visit you at home after the birth of your baby ensuring the health of both you and your baby. Depending on your birth experience or problems encountered the frequency may vary. But remember if staffing levels are low they may request that you come to them at the hospital/community setting for discharge. This will normally be on the tenth day providing your baby has regained birth weight and there are no problems for example, jaundice.

Before leaving the hospital you will be given a 'Red Book'. This is your baby's personal child health record book and is very important as it holds all the information you as a mother will need to know and it should be kept with you when you go for appointments with your baby. This is to provide you and the health professionals with up to date information on your child, for example, immunisation records. If you have not been given one the HV will bring one when she comes on her first visit. Once the midwife has discharged you and baby from her care the HV will take over the care. The HV will not usually turn up unannounced but one of her support team will normally phone and make an appointment. Sometimes the midwife and HV will overlap but it is rare.

Chapter One: Welcome to Parenthood

Health Visitor Input - New Birth Visit (7-14 day)

If you have not received an ante natal visit then this will be your first visit/new birth visit is normally lasts about an hour to an hour and a half. It will be divided into two distinct parts. Part one should focus on the baby and part two should focus on the mother. *(It is important to state that not all HVs will carry out a physical check of baby as many HVs do not now weigh the baby at home, thus will not have the opportunity to observe your baby. The following procedure is how I have been trained and my preferred way to practice).*

During this initial visit the HV will be giving you lots of information. This will be covered in detail in the next chapter. She should go through the 'red book' (otherwise known as my personal child held record) in detail with you so you are familiar with its contents.

She will give you contact numbers for herself and the team. It is important to note that health visiting is not an emergency service. They only work 9 to 5 Monday to Friday and of course things will always go wrong at the weekends or evenings. For anyone in need of help outside normal hours there is a 24hr helpline previously known as NHS direct you can contact them for advice on triple one (111).

The HV will go through lots of information with you about your own health and the health of your baby.

<u>Here is a sample of some of the information covered (it may vary depending on where you live):</u>

- Names and contact details of the health visiting team.
- Baby clinic information – where to find them and days and times.
- Breast feeding information.

Chapter One: Welcome to Parenthood

- Prevention of cot death information.
- Immunisation information.
- BCG leaflet.
- Children's centre information/registration form.
- Postnatal support groups.
- Vitamin D leaflet.

Mother

The HV will ask you about your birth experience as some research suggest that if a mother experiences a negative birth she may be more predisposed to getting depressed. I have to say that is not always true and was not my experience. I have known mothers to be depressed having had a very positive birth experience.

You will be asked about your health and your post-natal status:

- Breasts, sutures/stitches, lochia (Blood loss).
- Eating/Drinking
- Elimination- Bladder/Bowels
- Rest/Post natal exercises
- Cervical smear status
- Contraception/sexual health
- Post natal depression

Follow-up Visit

This visit will vary from 2 weeks to 6 weeks after the initial contact or new birth visit, or possibly not at all. You may be requested to just come to the baby clinic to see a HV and have your baby weighed. But if HV staff are in sufficient numbers or commissioners buy this service/key performance indicator (KPI) then this visit will be offered to you. Again, this visit will be conducted in two parts focussing on both baby and mother.

During this visit you can expect advice on the following:

- Feeding
- Sleeping
- Immunisations
- 6-8 week developmental check
- Post natal check/maternal mood assessment
- Any worries/concerns that you may have

This will probably be the last time you will see a HV in your home and all subsequent checks will be carried out by the support staff.

Developmental Assessments

6-8 week developmental check

As part of 'The Healthy Child Programme' (HCP) your baby will be offered a number of developmental screening examinations/assessments. The first one of these checks is at 6-8 weeks old. This is an important check carried out by the GP at your surgery. The GP should carry out a full physical check of your baby which includes:

- Height and weight check
- Heart and lungs – to check for any heart murmurs/defects
- Reflexes- Moro (startling), stepping etc.

Chapter One: Welcome to Parenthood

- Genitals
- Eyes/Ears
- Hips
- Rest of Body – fontanelle, palate, spine, abdomen etc.

8-12Mt Developmental Check

This developmental screening assessment is carried out by the health visiting service but may not be a HV, it could be a member of the skill mix team (Community Staff Nurse (CSN), Nursery Nurse (NN) or indeed a student HV). As well as carrying out height and weight measurements on your baby, the heath professional (HP) will ask lots of questions about the baby's health and development to get a clear picture of any deviations from normal. When assessing your baby the HP is looking at different areas of development.

The specific areas are:

- Communication
- Gross motor development
- Fine motor development
- Personal and Social development
- Problem Solving

In some areas they will send out a questionnaire for you to complete prior to inviting you for the check to get a better insight into your child's development. This is called an 'Ages and Stages Questionnaire' (ASQ) and then your child will be scored on their performance. It is important to be as honest as possible as they want to identify areas of weakness and refer your child for the specific help they may need, for example, speech and language therapy (SALT). Many parents want their child to score top marks, this is understandable but then your child may not get the support they need to develop and reach their full potential.

2-2.5yr Developmental Check

This is very similar to the above in format and follows the same approach. Some areas will carry out this check as a home visit; others will invite you to the clinic. This may be the last developmental check your child has before going to nursery or school so please ensure that you attend, as if you miss the opportunity your child may be disadvantaged if there is a problem with health or development. The health professional (HP) will always refer if there are concerns about your child or if you have any concerns about your child and call you back for a review. If everything is within normal limits at this check your child will not be offered the final check at 3.5yrs unless you are concerned.

Targeted 3.5yr check

This is mostly offered to children in the second and third category of health visiting caseloads. But if you have concerns or possibly missed your 2-2.5yr developmental check you can always request a check on your child.

Conclusion

The role of the HV is to advise, guide and support you through the first five years of your child's development. They are there for all the family to help you through birth to five years or until your child starts school. They are a valuable resource for you to use in helping to keep you and your family well in both mind and body. Please do use them if you have any concerns or worries, they will be glad to hear from you. Their main focus is to promote health and prevent ill health. Prevention is always better than cure. Early intervention is so important for good outcomes.

Having given you a brief overview of the role of the HV the next Chapter I will go into more detail about each individual visit.

Chapter Two - How to be Your own Health Visitor

Introduction

Let me state quite clearly that there is no substitute for seeing your HV in person and I would encourage all my readers to attend their own local child health clinic to have their baby weighed on a regular basis. This is the best indicator of the health of your baby. If you have any worries or concerns about your child, your HV can help.

That said it is a fact that many people do not use their health visiting service to its optimum. I am amazed at how many mothers do not take their babies to have regular weight checks. I am even more surprised that parents do not accept the invitation of HVs to have their child's developmental assessments carried out. This service is free to all parents and I feel parents are so privileged to have a service like this as there is no other country that offers this unique service. This provides an opportunity for you, the parent, to be given one to one time to discuss your child's development and growth. This is where any deviations from normal will be picked up and then the appropriate referral can be made. It is for this reason that I write this book to give all parents this vital information that you need to keep your baby healthy.

Background

Health visiting is 150 years old. When I trained as a HV back in 1990 the focus of the role of the HV was centred on four basic principles and they still hold true today.

1. The search for needs.

2. The stimulation of the awareness of health needs.

3. Influence of policies affecting health needs.

4. The facilitation of health-enhancing activities.

This is the prevention model that I have practised for 25 years in my role as a HV. I am passionate about the promotion of health and the prevention of ill-health. My three basic aims in this book are to:

- Prevent the occurrence of conditions or problems.
- Prevent the development of conditions or problems.
- Prevent the deterioration of established conditions or problems.

If this book can help you as parents to identify any concerns with your baby and seek medical advice then it will have served its purpose. Please use this book as a guide and if you have any concerns having read it go and see your HV or GP for a referral.

Post Birth Check (within 72 hrs of birth)

Your baby will have the first check by a paediatric doctor in the hospital after birth and you should not be discharged until this is completed. Included in this physical check is listening to your baby's heart and lungs. Checking the head, neck and spine for any abnormalities is important. Some babies can be born with spinal deformities like a small curvature or a minor form of Spina Bifida (where the spinal bones do not completely close) or hydrocephalus (water on the brain). I have nursed many babies born with these conditions in Ireland in the 1980s as it was not picked up back then. Taking folic acid and vitamins during pregnancy has significantly decreased this condition in newborns. More severe cases of this condition are now picked up during your antenatal scan so please do not worry. The doctor should assess your baby's reflexes - stepping, moro (startling) reflex.

Make sure the doctor examines inside your baby's' mouth to check for any deviations from normal (like cleft palate or tongue-tie) and behind the ears for skin tags which can be occasionally missed. Arms, legs, hips hands and feet including fingers and toes should be fully checked. Some babies can be born with an extra digit on either hands or feet. This is most common where the thumb or little finger is situated. Babies born by C- Section will have a routine scan of their hips to ensure that there is no problem following birth i.e. dislocation or subluxation of the hip joint. The ultrasound will check that the head of the femur (ball) has not slipped out of the socket joint.

Your baby should be fully undressed when examined by the doctor, this is to observe the buttocks and genitalia, in girls the – labia (lips) both external (majora) and internal (minora) and the presence of urethra (opening to the bladder) and vagina. In boys the scrotum should be checked for presence of both testes along with examination of the penis for any abnormalities. Some boys can be born with a deformity of the shaft of the penis with the opening of the penis occurring half way down the shaft or in more severe cases underneath the scrotum. This condition is called hypospadias, a rare but real occurrence. I am telling you about these conditions not to scare you but to arm you with information. As a sick children's nurse I have seen and nursed many children with various deviations from normal and the majority can be corrected.

It is also common for boys at birth to have testes high in the inguinal canal and sometimes refer to one or both testicles as being retractile – testicles can go up and down depending on temperature. If cold, testes tend to be high up and if hot they tend be down in the scrotum.

Tip # 1:

Best time to check for this is when taking the nappy off or when getting the baby out of the bath. This needs to be continually observed to prevent a problem with undescended testicles in the future. All results should be documented in your baby's hospital record for future reference and the outcome sent to your GP.

New birth Visit

The midwife will normally discharge you after the 10th day providing that your baby has regained birth weight and there are no problems with you or your baby. If your baby is premature or jaundiced this would be a reason for them to visit for a longer period. The HV will take over the health care needs after the midwife has discharged you and your baby. They will normally take the records with them, so if you want to keep a copy of your records I would suggest that you photocopy them.

The health visitor should carry out a home visit between days 7-14. This is a statutory visit that must be completed by day 14 at the latest. There are times when this target is not achieved, for example, when a mother moves in or out of an area just before the birth. It is important that you inform your midwife at the hospital if you are going to be discharged to a new address different from the address you gave when

Chapter Two: How to Be Your Own Health Visitor

you were booked at pregnancy. The HV will only have the information supplied to them by the hospital and sometimes this will be different. If your telephone number has changed it is also very useful to give the updated number to the hospital or midwife. The HV will again only act on the information given them on the birth notification from the hospital. If they have no contact number they will write to you but if the address and telephone number is wrong this will result in errors being made in administration.

In most cases the HV will try phoning to make an appointment with you before visiting and arrange a time that is suitable for you and your family. When she/he (male health visitors do exist but are rare) does visit they should introduce themselves and explain what the role of the HV is, as if this is your first baby you will not know. They will also explain about the 'red book'. The purpose of the red book is to enable you the mother to have all the information and knowledge you need about your baby until they reach school age (at that time the school nurse will take over the health care of your child). I will now take you through the red book step - by - step.

The red book is divided up into the following sections:

1. Child, family and birth details/local and information sources (Section one of red book, covered in this chapter)
2. Immunisation (Section two of red book - see chapter three in this book)
3. Screening and Routine Reviews (Section three of red book - already mentioned in chapter one)
4. Growth Charts (Section four of red book – see chapter six -clinics)

Birth Details and Newborn Examination

The HV will want to know about your birth experience. She will ask you the following:

- Place of birth (Hospital)
- Type of birth- SVD-spontaneous vaginal delivery, this can be with or without an episiotomy (a diagonal cut into the perineum to allow the baby to be born this will prevent a larger tear), C- Section (caesarean), forceps, ventouse also known as a vacuum (suction).
- Length of pregnancy –whether it was full term or premature.
- Any problems/complications with you or baby following delivery - infection or jaundice for example.
- Whether your baby was admitted to the neonatal unit.
- Whether your baby has had a Vitamin K injection this is routinely offered to all babies following birth to prevent bleeding.
- Newborn examination.
- Method of feeding- breast, bottle or mixed.

Physical Check of Baby

As a practising HV for over 20 years, I divide my new birth visit into two distinct parts. I first focus on the baby and then turn my focus to the mother. When I make an assessment of the baby I can only do so if I see the baby with my own eyes and to make a thorough assessment the baby needs to be seen naked. I work from head to toe in my assessment.

Head

Firstly, I look at the head shape of the head. Sometimes babies' heads can be affected by the type of birth experience they have had. If babies have had a difficult, long birth they can get a condition which is known as 'coning'. This is where the baby has been in the birth canal for a long period of time and the head has adopted that shape. Some parents get very concerned about this condition but there is no need to worry; the bones of the skull are very soft and soon the normal head shape will return.

If your baby has had a forceps delivery sometimes (but rarely) the forceps can leave marks either side of the head. Again these will quickly disappear. If your baby was born by ventouse then it is likely that they will also have a suction 'cap' shape over the top of the head. Please remember babies' heads are very soft and nature has made our babies in this way in order for them to fit through the birth canal. The bones will soon settle and resume a normal shape.

I always look at the fontanelle or 'soft spot' to see that it is what we like to see – 'normo-tensive'. This means that if you run your hand along the skull it is running in line with the rest of the skull shape. It should not be dipped or bulging. The fontanel tells you a lot about your baby. If it is dipped it can suggest that your baby is a little dry or dehydrated. It should not be looked at in isolation but as a complete picture.

By this I mean, if your baby is not drinking well and has dry nappies and if the fontanelle is dipped or sunken then these signs together would be worrying and you would need to take action to remedy the situation or your baby could become seriously ill. If, on the other hand, your baby's fontanelle is bulging and they are irritable or off their milk feeds, then they will need to see a doctor, it can be a sign of an underlying problem.

Eyes

Your baby's eyes should be clean and dry. Many babies are born with sticky eyes. During birth when passing through the birth canal they can pick up minor irritations or infections. 99% of them will resolve with just swabbing with cool boiled water. There are natural healing properties in breast milk so if you are breastfeeding you can swab with breast milk. If the eyes continue to be sticky it is not a concern it will only be a problem if the white of the eye becomes red or bloodshot looking. This is called 'conjunctivitis' and will need treatment with antibiotics. Sometimes, discharge of a watery substance can persist and on rare occasions the baby can have a blocked lacrimal/tear duct. This may get better as the baby grows, so will their ducts. If this does not resolve by a year old your GP will refer to have the ducts probed to unblock them. You can help the drainage of tears by gently massaging the duct just under the eye to the side of the nose on the inner aspect of the eye.

The other condition that babies' sometimes get is yellow discolouration in the eyes - a mild form of jaundice, this also is evident in the skin.

Jaundice

Jaundice is the name given to the yellow appearance of the skin and whites of the eye. Jaundice is common in newborn babies and occurs in about 90% of babies. When your baby is in the womb all the waste products are taken away by the placenta. After birth, the baby has to do this for himself and it can take a little longer. One of the waste products is bilirubin this is the end product of red blood cells when they are broken down. It's normal for red cells to be broken down as we continuously make new ones (the cycle takes 120 days from

Chapter Two: How to Be Your Own Health Visitor

beginning to end in adults shorter for newborns). The liver is the organ responsible for breaking down the excess and this can be a little slow at first, that's why it can sometimes build up in the beginning.

Jaundice will normally appear around day two or three and reach its peak at day 4 or 5. This is known as physiological jaundice of the newborn and will resolve on its own normally about day 10-14. Your baby will not be ill in anyway. We will ask you to feed more often as passing more urine will help, along with placing your baby near sunlight, like a window for example. Be careful not to burn your baby from the direct sunlight.

You can do the following measures and monitor the situation. You should check the colour of your baby's stool and urine. The stools of a breastfed baby should be greenish or daffodil yellow. The stools of a bottle fed baby should be greenish and mustard yellow. The urine should be colourless.

If your midwife is worried she will take a blood test from the heel to see what the level is and in rare cases your baby may have to return to hospital for some phototherapy to help the process along. This involves being placed in an incubator with strong ultraviolet light directly on your baby. Their eyes will be protected with a mask.

If the jaundice is persistent and you are worried contact your midwife, GP or HV if your midwife has discharged you. Some babies will remain jaundiced, here are a few reasons why:

If your baby is premature it will take longer for jaundice to resolve.

Your baby may have an underlying condition and should be referred to a GP who in turn will refer to a paediatric haematologist (blood) doctor.

Sometimes it persists a little longer in a breastfeeding baby.

Your baby may have an infection or other illness.

Your baby may have a thyroid problem but this is tested for on day 5 known as the PKU or blood spot test.

Your baby may have a problem with their liver but this is rare.

Golden Rule:

If your baby continues to have jaundice beyond 14 days in a full term baby or 21 days in a premature baby then you should have it investigated.

If your baby's stools or urine are not the right colour regardless of how old your baby is don't wait, have it investigated. Most clinics will have a stool chart so you can make a comparison. If not email:info@childliverdisease.org/www.childliverdisease.org

Nose

Your baby is born with very small nasal passages and if they have had a C- Section they are sometimes more prone to having mucus and being snuffly. It can be made worse by air conditioning in the home. As what happens is their mucus dries in the nasal passages and the baby can't really breathe as effectively with partial blockages. The mucus becomes dry and hard like 'bogies' but of course babies' can't pick their noses like adults can. Sometimes this can interfere with feeding as when the baby feeds the baby needs his/her nose to breathe through as the mouth is effectively blocked off. You can help ease breathing if giving the baby some saline (salt water) nose drops. These can be bought over the counter without prescription. Place 1 drop into each nostril before a feed and it will help to loosen the hard mucus/bogies and your baby will either sneeze them out or they will loosen and your baby may swallow it. Don't worry, it won't do them any harm it may make their stools a little loose but no harm will come to them.

Tip # 2:

Try and have a bowl of water in your home over the radiators as this will help to humidify the dry air.

Mouth

Try and get in the habit of checking your baby's mouth before or after feeding. A good opportunity to do this is when they are crying rather than force the mouth open. The tongue of a breastfed baby is usually coated with milk this is normal. Some babies are prone to oral thrush especially if they have been on antibiotics in hospital. However, some babies can pick up thrush from the mother but only if breastfeeding, as it is transferred from the nipple to the mucus membrane in the baby's mouth. Thrush is a fungal infection and in order for thrush to grow it needs three conditions; food, moisture and heat. The breastfeeding mother's nipples are a perfect breeding ground for thrush to occur. It is easy to overlook but it is recognised in the mother by a pin prick rash on the areola (pigmented part of the nipple) and sometimes accompanied by an itching and sharp shooting pain but not always. The infection is then transferred to the baby's mouth. It is recognised in the baby by white elevated patches. It will normally start on the inside of the mouth on the sides and then it transfers to the roof of the mouth and lastly the tongue. It can be painful and will stop the baby from sucking. The treatment is an antifungal cream. The medication of choice from GPs is Nystatin oral suspension. GPs tend to prescribe this as a first line of treatment.

I find that this is not always effective and results are better with Daktarin oral gel. The mother must also be treated or else the condition will re-occur. The treatment for the mother is Daktarin cream. The cream is available without prescription however; the oral gel for baby no longer is available over the counter it has to be obtained by prescription.

Tongue-Tie

Some babies are born with a tight piece of skin called the 'frenulum' between the underside of their tongue and the floor of the mouth. This can vary in severity from very minor to complete tethering of the tongue which will make it very difficult for the baby to feed effectively. Most babies will not need intervention but if your baby is experiencing difficulty with feeding then it is best to have it snipped to loosen the tongue. Unfortunately you will not be referred until your baby experiences feeding problems, which is a shame. My advice is to go to your breastfeeding cafe and speak with a breastfeeding advisor and they sometimes have the authority to refer you. If you do not have a breastfeeding cafe near to you go and see your GP who will refer you to your nearest hospital to have the procedure carried out.

Skin

It is important to get a good overview of the baby's skin as a whole. I always ask about the condition of the skin, many babies who are overdue will have dry skin especially around the wrists and ankles. It is good to oil your baby if they are peeling. Bathing will tend to dry your baby's skin out more especially if you live in a hard water area like London. Many parents are tempted to bath their babies' every day, which is not necessary.

I always look for birth marks on babies' as they are very common. Different cultures will have different birth marks for example 'blue spot' birth marks are common in Afro-Caribbean and Asian cultures. They are predominantly found over the cheeks of the buttocks or around the small of the back. However, they can also be found on the limbs or hands/feet, rarely on the abdomen or back. Whereas, 'stork' marks and 'strawberry' marks, are more common in white Caucasian families. Stork marks are predominantly found between the eyes on the forehead, or at the back of the neck. They are light in colour but when the baby cries they become darker in colour. 'Strawberry' marks can be found anywhere on the body. The majority of 'strawberry' marks get bigger in size in the first year and then 90% will disappear after the age of nine years. Port-wine stains are purple-red in colour usually bigger in size. These seldom fade with age, but can be treated with laser. It is best to carry out this procedure after the age of seventeen.

Nappy area

Newborn babies rarely get nappy rash but in some circumstances it can appear. If you or your baby has been on antibiotics this will give your baby loose stools which will in turn make your baby's skin sore around the nappy area. It is of course important to avoid nappy rash by frequent changing of soiled nappies. But even despite this sometimes your baby will still get sore.

Tip # 3:

When your baby has nappy rash avoid baby wipes and use water and cotton wool instead. This will help your baby to heal. Only use wipes when you are away from home. Try to avoid regular use of creams like sudocrem only use when needed.

There are a number of creams on the market to help with nappy rash my recommendation is Metanium ointment. It can be bought over the counter no prescription needed. It will act as a barrier and help heal the skin from inside out. Please note that the skin will take up the yellowness of the cream do not try and wash hard to get if off you will damage the skin. But instead use oil (olive/almond) which will remove the old stale cream without damage to the skin.

Circumcision

In some cultures it is customary to perform a circumcision in boys. This will usually be carried out within the first couple of weeks by trained professional or doctor who has been trained to perform the procedure. This procedure is not carried out under the NHS and will only be done for medical reasons. It is important that you find someone who is qualified to undertake this procedure to prevent any complications occurring. Of course, even with qualified and competent practitioners some babies will still get minor complications for example, bleeding or infection. You will need to consult a GP if concerned.

Nails

Just a note about finger and toe nails many parents worry about cutting their baby's nails. Please don't bite your baby's nails as you can introduce infections and result in a condition called Paronychia. This is when the nail bed becomes red warm, tender and swollen along the edge of the nail. It is best to buy a baby nail clippers and clip when the nails are soft like after a bath. If you notice any signs of infection in the nail please go and see your GP your baby may need antibiotics.

This completes the physical check of baby. The role of the HV is to prevent ill-health and promote health. This visit is the most important time to talk about the prevention of cot death. See next page.

Milk Spots (milia)

Your baby is likely to have milia, which is common in newborns. Tiny, white spots appear, usually across the nose, cheeks, chin, forehead or around the eyes. Milia look raised, but if you touch them they will feel smooth.

Milia normally appear a couple of weeks after birth because the oil glands on your baby's face are still developing. Your baby's milia spots should clear up on their own within a month or six weeks.

Heat Rash

If your baby suddenly develops a bright-red pimply rash on his neck, under his arms, or near the edges of his nappy or underwear, it's probably heat rash. Heat rash, also known as prickly heat can appear when your baby overheats in hot and humid weather.

The rash often appears in folds of your baby's skin and on parts of his body where clothing fits snugly. If your baby wears hats, the rash may even spread across his scalp or forehead. Make sure your baby wears natural fibres next to the skin (cotton) as this will allow the skin to breathe, avoid synthetic fibres like polyester or nylon.

Prevention of Cot Death/Sudden Infant Death Syndrome (SIDS)

This is the sudden and unexpected death of an infant. Every year in the UK 300 babies will die unexpectedly.

As part of the HVs physical checks it is good practice to teach the parents about the prevention of cot death. This involves having both the baby's temperature and room temperature comfortable for the baby. Temperature regulation is an important factor in the prevention of cot death and how to assess your baby's temperature. It is important that parents feel central 'core' temperature – back of neck, tummy or chest. Hands and feet will always be colder to the touch and many parents make the mistake of assessing peripherals (hands and feet) instead of 'core' temperature and can sometimes overheat a baby by putting on another layer of clothing or an extra blanket.

I have only seen two cots deaths in my 30yrs as a professional so thankfully it is rare, but devastating if it happens to you and your family. So prevention is so important. We do not know the reason behind cot death but we do know that there are some factors that contribute to cot death.

What can I do to help prevent SIDS?

Follow the advice below to help prevent SIDS:

- Place your baby on their back to sleep, in a cot in the room with you.
- Don't smoke during pregnancy or let anyone smoke in the same room as your baby.
- Don't share a bed with your baby if you or your partner smoke or take drugs, or if you have been drinking alcohol.

Chapter Two: How to Be Your Own Health Visitor

- Never sleep with your baby on a sofa or armchair.
- Don't let your baby get too hot or too cold.
- Keep your baby's head uncovered. Their blanket should be tucked in no higher than their shoulders.
- Place your baby in the "feet to foot" position (with their feet touching the end of the cot or pram).
- If possible, breastfeed your baby.

Tip # 4:
Always make sure your baby has natural fibres next to its skin, like cotton. Blankets should be cellular or cotton (when you hold the blanket towards the window you should be able to see sunlight through them). This means the skin can breathe. Avoid any man-made fibres like nylon or polyester, they trap air and overheat your baby. Baby duvets and sleep suits/nests look pretty but can be dangerous if they are not made of natural fibres.

If feeding in bed at night always place your baby back into their own crib/cot as your duvet will be too hot for a baby.

Chapter Three - Immunisations

Childhood Immunisation Programme

The immunisation programme is a universal programme that is offered to all babies by the Department of Health (DOH). Each country will have their own programme with slight variations. There will also be some regional variations, for example, in London all babies born in high risk areas will be offered the BCG injection against tuberculosis (TB). The reason behind this is that in London there is a higher incidence of TB than in other parts of the country. The reason behind this is wherever you have built-up areas with many people living in close proximity there is more risk of transmission. To prevent a spread of this disease it is safer and cheaper for the DOH to prevent the disease.

Immunisations

In July 2013 the government introduced changes to the immunisation programme. There will now be an additional oral vaccine to protect against Rotavirus. This is a serious and infectious form of gastroenteritis (diarrhoea and vomiting). The majority of Trusts set down what the Department of Health advises with the exception of BCG- Bacillus Calmette- Guerin. Some Trusts will vary in whether they offer BCG vaccination to prevent TB, as not everyone will be susceptible to it, (you are more at risk if living in inner cities and London is a high risk area). This is not available from your GP and can be only taken up in a community based clinic as the funding is not available to GPs.

Chapter Three: Immunisations

What is BCG Vaccine?

The BCG is a live vaccine that contains a weakened form of the bacteria that cause TB. Because it is a weakened form of the disease your baby will not develop TB but produce antibodies to fight against the disease if your baby should come into contact with TB.

What is TB?

TB is a serious infectious disease that affects the lungs, but it can also affect the brain, glands and bones. If the brain is affected you can suffer from a condition called TB meningitis. The treatment is long and takes several months but most people will make a full recovery from the disease.

How is it transferred?

You can only catch TB from someone whose lungs or throat have already got the infection. When they cough they will spray the droplets into the air and they are then inhaled into your baby. The droplets can stay in the air for quite long periods of time. But you will need to have prolonged close exposure to someone who is infected to pick up the disease.

Symptoms

- A cough that lasts longer than three weeks/coughing up blood

Chapter Three: Immunisations

- A fever/high temperature
- Night sweats
- Weight loss
- Feeling tired

How is my Baby Immunised?

Your baby will be given the injection just under the skin surface in the left upper arm. It is universally recognised as it will leave a scar.

Side Effects

Immediately after the injection a blister will appear (but not always), this is a sign that the injection has been given properly i.e. just under the skin.

Within 2-6 weeks after having the injection a small spot will appear (but again not always so don't worry babies will react differently). It may be quite sore to touch and your baby may be a little irritable. The spot should gradually heal. In some cases the spot may fill with pus and burst, oozing fluid. In this case just cover with a dry bandage and avoid putting a plaster on. This sore may take several months to heal. If worried consult your GP or HV.

The primary immunisations will, however, be available at both your local baby clinic/GP surgery at 8, 12 and 16 weeks of age. These include:

Chapter Three: Immunisations

8 Weeks – DTap/IPV/HIB PCV and Rotavirus

Two Injections

Injection 1- Diphtheria, Tetanus, acelluar Pertussis (whooping cough), Inactivated Polio Vaccine, Haemophilus influenza b (HIB)

Injection 2- Pneumococcal (PCV)

Rotavirus given orally

12 Weeks – DTap/IPV/HIB, Men C and Rotavirus

Two Injections

Injection 1 - Diphtheria, Tetanus, Pertussis (whooping cough), Haemophilus influenza b (HIB)

Injection 2- Meningococcal C (Men C)

Rotavirus given orally

16 Weeks – DTap/IPV/HIB, Men C and PVC

Two Injections

Injection 1- Diphtheria, Tetanus, Pertussis (whooping cough) Haemophilus influenza b (HIB)

Injection 2 – Pneumococcal (PCV)

12mts

Three Injections

Injection 1- Measles, Mumps, Rubella (MMR)

Injection 2 - Haemophilus influenza b (HIB) and Meningococcal C

Injection 3 – Pneumococcal (PCV)

Chapter Three: Immunisations

15mts -MMR

One Injection

Measles, Mumps and Rubella (MMR)

3 Years and Four Months and Over – DTap/IPV or dTaP/IPV

One Injection

Injection 1- Diphtheria or low dose diphtheria, Tetanus, Pertussis, Inactivated Polio Vaccine preschool booster.

NOTE: All immunisations should be booked at your GP surgery by appointment or you can just drop into your local child health clinic (no appointment needed but you will be waiting for longer).

* All information correct at time of going to press

What is Diphtheria?

Diphtheria is a serious disease that usually begins in the throat with soreness and then quickly can lead to breathing problems. It can damage the heart and nervous system and in severe cases, it can kill.

What is Tetanus?

Tetanus is a disease affecting the nervous system which can lead to muscle spasm, causing breathing problems and can kill. It is caused

Chapter Three: Immunisations

when bacteria which can be present in soil and manure this can gets into the body through open cuts or burns.

What is Pertussis (Whooping Cough)?

Whooping cough is a disease that can cause long bouts of coughing and choking, making it hard to breathe. Whooping Cough can last for up to 10 weeks. Babies under one year of age are most at risk from Whooping Cough.

In 2013 there was an outbreak of Whopping Cough and 10 babies in California died as a result. The government (DOH) responded by offering all pregnant women the immunisation in late pregnancy to protect their unborn baby as the vaccine is not given until your baby is 8 weeks old.

What is Polio?

Polio is a virus that attacks the nervous system and can cause permanent paralysis of muscles. If it affects the chest muscles or the brain, Polio can kill.

What is Rotavirus?

Rotavirus is a particularly contagious form of diarrhoea affecting young babies (seen mostly in hospitals where sick babies are more at risk due lower immunity but can also be seen in the community).

What is Hib?

Hib is an infection caused by Haemophilus influenza type b bacteria. It can lead to a number of major illnesses such as blood poisoning

(Septicaemia), Pneumonia and Meningitis. It only protects against the type b strain of Meningitis. There are, of course, other strains hence the government adding Meningitis C to the immunisation programme.

What is Pneumococcal Vaccine?

Pneumococcal infection is one of the commonest causes of Meningitis but it also causes ear infections, Pneumonia and some other serious illnesses.

What is Meningococcal C?

This vaccine protects against Meningitis and Septicaemia (blood poisoning) caused by the 'Meningococcal group C' bacteria.

MMR Vaccine (Measles, Mumps and Rubella)

What is Measles?

Measles is caused by a viral infection which is very contagious. Nearly everyone who catches measles will have a high temperature, a rash and generally be unwell. Children will be in bed for about 5 to 10 days and off school. Adults are likely to be ill for longer. The complications of measles affect about 1 in every 15 children and can include the following:

- Chest infections
- Fits
- Ear infections (in severe cases deafness)

- Blood infections
- Brain infections – Encephalitis
- Death

What is Mumps?

Mumps is caused by a virus which can lead to a high temperature, headache, and painful swelling of the glands in the face, neck and jaw. It can result in permanent deafness, viral Meningitis and Encephalitis. In males it can lead to swelling in the testicles, in rare cases it can lead to sterility. It also affects the ovaries in females.

What is Rubella?

Rubella or German measles is also caused by a virus. In children it is usually mild and can go unnoticed. It causes a short-lived rash, swollen glands and a sore throat. Rubella is very serious in unborn babies. It can seriously damage the following:

- Sight
- Hearing
- Heart
- Brain

This condition is called Congenital Rubella Syndrome (CRS). Contact with rubella within the first three months of pregnancy will lead to damage to the unborn baby in nine out of ten cases.

Chapter Three: Immunisations

Advice to Parents after Your Child Has Been Immunised

Most babies and children will have no ill effects after their immunisations. A few children do have minor reactions but nearly all can be dealt with by the parent. You will rarely need medical intervention.

General Reactions

Sometimes your baby will be a bit grumpy and irritable, this happens quite often, but does not last long. Try distracting your baby with cuddles, toys or drinks.

Persistent Crying or Screaming

Contact your GP or HV if in doubt. If you are unable to contact a health professional then contact the NHS helpline of 111 (this is a 24hr helpline available for all the family) They will advise you if you need to go to A&E for help.

Prolonged Severe Fever

The quickest way to bring down a baby's fever is to remove his/her clothes and give cool drinks. If this doesn't work then sponge them down with lukewarm water (not cold). You can give infant paracetamol. The dose to give will be on the bottle. For babies under 3 months of age, it is not usually recommended. *However, following immunisation, even if your baby is less than 3 months old, you may give your child infant paracetamol.*

NB The dose of 60mgs which is 2.5mls (half a teaspoon) of infant paracetamol suspension may be given. This can be repeated ONCE after 4 hours only.

If after this intervention your baby has still got a high temperature then consult a GP/HV/A&E.

Convulsions or Fits

Very occasionally these can occur in babies with a very high temperature usually over 40 degrees Celsius. Normal body temperature is between 36-37 degrees Celsius.

If this happens make sure your baby is in a safe place on a flat surface. Place them on their tummy with the head to one side. Do not put anything in the mouth. Stay with your baby until the fit is over it will only last a minute (but will seem like an eternity to you) then call for an ambulance. A fit is nature's way of bringing down a high temperature, so always try and keep a check on this to avoid it happening.

Local Reactions

These include: slight redness or swelling around the injection site, up to the size of a 10p piece is acceptable reaction. Sometimes a hard lump forms under the skin. This is caused by the baby sometimes moving away during the needle going in; this results in the fluid infiltrating into the tissues rather than the muscle. To avoid this try and hold your baby's body tight with their arm immobilised during the procedure to avoid them pulling away. Both of these minor problems will disappear without treatment.

Any redness or swelling, which is more than 3inches (7cm) across should be bought to the attention of the GP.

Rashes

After 7-10 days of having the MMR immunisation, the child can feel unwell, develop a high temperature and a mild rash may appear. This is the modified measles' reaction. It is not severe and is not infectious. Apart from reducing the temperature, no special treatment is required.

After 2-3 weeks of having the MMR immunisation, babies can occasionally (in 1% of cases) get slightly swollen neck glands. This is the mumps component of the vaccine taking effect.

Tip # 6:

How to detect a meningitis rash (red blotches on skin)

The 'Glass Test' – Press the side of a clear drinking glass firmly against the rash so you can see if the rash fades or loses colour under pressure. If it doesn't change colour contact your GP or go to the hospital immediately.

NOTE:

In Feb 1998, Dr Andrew Wakefield published a 12 patient study in the medical journal 'The Lancet'. He proposed a link with the MMR and a 'new syndrome' of autism and bowel disease. Wakefield urged the parents to use single vaccine instead of MMR.

After this scare the numbers of parents taking up the vaccine dropped and continued to drop. Many private clinics opened up offering single doses of Measles, Mumps and Rubella.

Chapter Three: Immunisations

In 2006 the UK saw the first death from measles in 14years.

In 2010 Wakefield was found guilty of serious professional misconduct and his name was removed from the medical register.

However, the effects were long lasting and in 2013 in South West Wales there was an epidemic of Measles with over 1,200 cases reported and sadly another death from Measles.

We are now almost 20yrs on from that research being carried out and are still suffering from its effects, I still get parents choosing not to immunise their children.

Chapter Four – Maternal Health and Well Being

General Advice Given to Parent at New Birth Visit

There is so much administration to carry out and appointments to attend once you have had a baby it can feel a bit overwhelming. So it is important that your partner/husband be available to help you with this.

Registration of Birth and with GP

Every baby needs to be registered by day 42 at the local authority birth registration department in whichever borough the baby was born. Most hospitals will give you the information needed to register your baby, before you leave the hospital. If they don't give you this information then ASK them. If you are married you can get your husband to register the birth without you being present.

If you are not married, then both of you must go to register the birth together. If you are a single mother you need to think carefully about whether you put the name of the father on the birth certificate or not as there will be implications for you and your baby.

If you choose to put the father's name on the birth certificate this means that your partner has parental responsibility. What does that imply? Well, it means that if you and your partner ever break up he has an equal right or 'say' in what happens with your child. This could be minor things like whether he/she can have their hair cut, to what school they go to, or in extreme cases, even whether you can take them out of the country. This is the law and the absent parent, whether it be the mother or the father, are within their rights to have their 'say'. He/she will also have the right to access, visitation and holiday time with your children- even if there is a history of abuse. However, the access may be supervised usually by a family member or in a local authority setting depending on the circumstances, but not always. This many see as a negative. Please don't get me wrong I think it is important for a child to have both parents in their lives as long as it keeps the child safe and there is no risk of harm.

However, the upside of naming the father on the birth certificate is that parental responsibility also means taking responsibility for the financial cost of raising a child. If you and your partner go your separate ways then your partner has the legal obligation to provide for their child financially. All that the residing parent (usually the mother but not always) has to do is give the name of the absent parent to the CSA (Child Support Agency) and they will track them down and make them pay maintenance for the baby. The money will be taken directly out of their bank account and transferred into yours, providing they are working of course, but even if they are not working they will be in receipt of government benefits and they will normally still have to pay a small amount towards the cost of raising the baby.

If a mother decides not to name the father he can still get access to his baby through the courts. I am not biased towards either parent as long as the parenting on both sides is positive.

How Can the Birth Father Voluntarily Establish Paternity?

If a father wants to formally establish paternity, he should begin by voluntarily acknowledging paternity. In doing so, he agrees to accept responsibility for the child and pay child support until the child reaches the age of majority.

The birth father can voluntarily acknowledge paternity in two ways:

Chapter Four: Maternal Health and Well Being

Firstly, he can be present at the birth of the child and sign a Declaration of Paternity. (Sometimes this paperwork is called an Acknowledgment of Paternity.) This documentation is also necessary in order to have a father's name placed on the child's birth certificate, if you choose to do so.

Secondly, if he is not present at the birth, he can complete an affidavit of paternity any time between the birth of the child up until the child turns 18. If this document is not completed before the birth certificate is issued, and you want the father's name listed on the birth certificate, you can apply to have the birth certificate altered to add the father's name at a later date.

Once you get the birth registered you will then need to register with GP. If you are staying with the same GP then this is usually straight forward just bring your 'red book' and get the registration forms. If you decide to go to a new GP they will want to see a copy of the birth certificate in order to register your baby, especially if you are not known to that surgery. This is a precaution to ensure that the baby is yours and has been delivered in this country. Some babies are born outside of the UK and although the NHS provides treatment to all at point of entry it is important that every baby is known and registered for record keeping purposes as some families will not be entitled to other services/benefits if they do not live within the EU. Many families will of course come as refugees or asylum seekers into the country and others will gain entry illegally.

Once you present the birth certificate your baby will then be registered with the GP and be given access to services. Your baby will already have been given a unique National Health Service (NHS) number by the hospital after birth.

Chapter Four: Maternal Health and Well Being

Benefits

Once you have received your child's birth certificate you can then send off for your Child Benefit. This was a universal benefit to all children born in the UK. But recently in 2013 the regulations on this changed and now if you are a high earner (you or your partner earns over £50,000) you will no longer be entitled to this benefit. Please visit this website www.moneyadviceservice.co.uk for full information. If you earn below this amount this is what the rates will be based on rates July 2013:

Basic weekly amount:

First Child - £20.50

Second child - £13.55

Subsequent children - £13.55

If you are a UK citizen and are unemployed or a student you will be entitled to other benefits like income support, family tax credit and housing benefits. However, I am not a benefits expert so please consult the web address I gave you earlier or seek independent advice from your Citizens Advice Bureau.

Physical Assessment of Mother

Having a baby is a major life even and it can take its toll on your body, some will sail through the labour and delivery others will experience much difficulty. I must admit that I felt awful after the birth of my first baby. Breastfeeding did not come naturally to me and I struggled. My stitches were tight and uncomfortable - I also had painful haemorrhoids (piles) from pushing. Here is an account of my personal experience.

Personal Story

After Ben (my first baby) was born I knew the importance of skin to skin contact so I put him to the breast straight away. He wasn't that interested in sucking as he was exhausted from a long drawn out labour.

After delivery we were put in a side room and I didn't see any midwife until the next morning. I had tried to breastfeed Ben in the night without success. He had passed urine (wee) and meconium (poo) so we were discharged home after the doctor had checked him over. He still had not had a feed; he just simply messed about at the nipple, never really getting a good enough latch. By now my milk had come in and my boobs were like melons- big, round and hard. I started expressing to relieve the pressure and gave the milk to Ben by cup and spoon as I did not want to give him 'nipple confusion'. The midwife came the next day and I thought, thank god she will help me, but she came and went. Her only advice was to preserve.

Chapter Four: Maternal Health and Well Being

By the time she came back on day 5 my nipples were cracked and bleeding, he still hadn't managed to have a proper feed. I was now in a desperate state. I saw a different midwife this time and thought I might get some help. She suggested putting 'savoy' cabbage leaves in the freezer and then placing them inside my bra; I was so desperate that I would have tried anything to try soothing the pain. When she left I burst into tears, I didn't want to give up as I didn't want to be a failure. (I couldn't after all I was a health visitor).

By day 7 I had developed mastitis (infection in the breast ducts) and was so ill I couldn't function properly. I eventually managed to get Ben breastfeeding successfully but only through sheer determination and lots of hard work. I have to say that breastfeeding was, for me it was one of the hardest but most rewarding experiences of being a mother and I totally loved it - eventually. I carried on feeding him until he was 12 months old and by then I was 2 months pregnant with my second baby. I probably would have continued had I not been so tired.

Many women don't get the support or information they need to be successful in their breastfeeding. Many women ask me how do I know if my baby is getting enough breast milk?

The following guidance is based on a baby in or around day 5.

1. Urinary output

If your baby is having at least 5-6 heavy wet nappies in 24 hours this is a good indication.

2. Baby's colour, alertness and tone.

Chapter Four: Maternal Health and Well Being

Your baby should have normal skin colour, alert and have good tone (not dry.)

3. Weight (following initial post-birth weight loss)

When your baby is re-weighed they should not have lost more than 10% of birth weight.

4. Number of feeds in 24hrs

At least 8 feeds in a 24 hour period.

5. Sucking pattern during a feed

Your baby should draw the nipple back to the soft palate at the back of the throat and initial suck with rapid sucks, then change to slower sucks with pauses and soft swallowing.

6. Length of feed

Baby will feed for 5-30mins. Sometimes baby will just be thirsty and take the foremilk (thinner milk with less fat), in order to get the hind milk (fattier milk) they will need to stay on for 20-30mins. A baby staying on for longer than 40mins or less than 5 minutes is concerning.

7. End of feed

Your baby should let go spontaneously when full, it is important not to take them off before they are ready to do so.

8. Offer the second breast

Some babies will want the second breast others will not, it depends on appetite.

9. Baby's behaviour after feeding

Chapter Four: Maternal Health and Well Being

Your baby should be happy, content and settled after a feed. If your baby is not settled seek help.

10. Shape of nipple after feed

The nipple should be the same shape as when the feed began or slightly elongated. If the nipple is misshapen or pinched at the end of a feed, again seek help.

11. Self-Reporting

After a feed the nipples and breast should be comfortable. If the nipples or breast are sore this could mean an underlying problem- engorgement/mastitis. Seek medical help.

Breast care

If you do not breast feed, your breasts will become quite hard as the milk comes in. It is more comfortable if you wear a good supporting bra and take regular painkillers like paracetamol. When you are breastfeeding it is very important for you to eat and drink well. You will find that you will be very thirsty as most of the fluid you drink will go into making your breast milk. If you do not drink enough you will become dehydrated and may suffer from headaches, cystitis, urinary tract infections, piles and constipation. These all result from not having sufficient fluids. Try to avoid this by increasing your fluid intake. All breastfeeding mothers should be on vitamin supplements.

Tip # 7:

I also recommend an iron supplement as breastfeeding is exhausting. You can buy supplements in your local pharmacy like 'Spa Tone Iron' or in your local supermarket like 'Fluradix'. These will give you a little bit more energy.

Many mothers give up on breastfeeding as they sadly feel that they don't get the right support or the correct information needed to succeed. Breastfeeding isn't easy, as you know I found it very hard indeed.

Here are my top tips to successful breastfeeding.

Common Problems

1. Sore nipples - this is unavoidable in the early days as the nipples are not used to such aggressive sucking. Your nipples will get tougher and soon this soreness will pass as long as you are positioning your baby correctly on the breast. There are creams that will ease the soreness but it will not magically disappear, time is the best healer.

2. Cracked nipples - This is caused by incorrect positioning. Your baby must suck your nipple with the soft palate at the back of the throat. If your baby does not draw the nipple in far enough they will suck with the hard palate at the front, this is what causes the nipple to crack. To correct this please draw as much of the nipple towards the back of the baby's mouth. Do not allow your baby to suck if it is painful after the first few sucks, this means that the position is wrong.

3. Thrush – I have mentioned this before but always ensure to treat both yourself and your baby.

4. Mastitis – this is where the breast has become infected with a bacterial infection but can also be caused by hormonal changes leading to too much milk being produced, a common occurrence in the first month. Sometimes, if the nipples are cracked an infection can be

introduced that way. If the breast becomes red swollen and tender, you will also feel unwell with flu like symptoms. Consult a doctor as you will need antibiotics to get rid of the infection.

5. Engorgement - This is where the milk ducts become over full, normally if your baby does not feed for a long time i.e. overnight or if you have given a bottle feed for whatever reason. The breast will become engorged with milk. It is important to get these milk ducts emptied as if left to build up it can also lead to mastitis. Some women will express to relive the discomfort others will manually express the milk by getting in a bath and placing hot flannel over the breast to get the milk flowing. The best way to relieve it is to get your baby to feed.

5. Nipple vasospasm or Raynaud's phenomenon) – is the condition where blood flow to the nipples is reduced, abruptly and leads to blanching of the nipple, and possible nipple colour changes to purple or blue. This tends to occur in thin women with poor circulation, who have a family history of Raynaud's phenomenon in the fingers. The pain is worsened by the cold, so the most effective step is to keep the nipples warm. If this is a problem for you go to your GP for treatment (Nifedipine is the drug normally prescribed).

Knowing these common problems is important as this knowledge can help you to avoid them. Get it right from the beginning and you prevent the above problems hopefully. Here is my advice if you wish to avoid problems for you and your baby.

Initiating Breastfeeding/Skin-to-Skin Contact/Rooming-in

Immediately after the baby is born best practice is to have skin-to-skin contact and to have your baby close to you. This way both of you will benefit from the hormonal effects of nature.

Chapter Four: Maternal Health and Well Being

The advantages of this for you;

It will stimulate your breastfeeding hormone 'prolactin' as this is triggered by touch (skin contact in the early weeks will result in prolactin surges which will help to sustain breastfeeding in the longer term). The closeness of you and your baby will also stimulate another hormone called 'oxytocin' which will calm you, much needed after birth especially if it is prolonged labour or a not so straight forward birth.

The advantages to your baby:

This will counteract the birth experience.

Your baby will be relaxed and produce the hormone 'adrenaline'.

They will start to root for the breast and this will stimulate your baby's digestion, even if they don't feed it will still start the progress.

It will help regulate the heart beat and breathing.

Skin-to-skin contact will help regulate the body temperature.

Baby is colonised by your skin bacteria which he/she will be exposed to when at home (don't worry this is 'friendly' bacteria but if any is not so friendly then your antibodies in the milk will fight against it).

Baby is stimulated by your touch and smell and a series of pre-feeding behaviours begin. These inborn reflexes only happen when close to you.

<u>For more information on initiating breastfeeding go to</u> http://www.unicef.org.uk.

NOTE: I know there will be many of you mothers reading this that have not had the benefit of 'rooming-in' (this means your baby staying with

Chapter Four: Maternal Health and Well Being

you from birth) for whatever reason, maybe your baby had to go to N.I.C.U (neonatal intensive care unit) for example.

I know this because I was one of these mothers. The good thing is that it is never too late to start breastfeeding. If breastfeeding has not got off to a good start then 'begin again' with skin-to-skin contact. You can get help and supports from many agencies just ask your health visitor about their baby feeding cafes/support groups there will be breastfeeding advisors in most areas where you live. Please see the list at the back of this book for other agencies that can help you.

Hand Expression – to express milk the milk (lactiferous) ducts will need to be compressed. This is achieved by making a 'C' shape with your thumb and the rest of your fingers about an inch behind the nipple. Gently squeeze then release finding your own rhythm.

If you are unable to breast fed in the early days like me. You may have to cup and spoon feed your baby if your baby is unable to latch onto the breast. Hand expression is the ideal method of expressing milk in the first few days for the following reasons:

Colostrum which is low in volume may get lost in the pump.

Milk expressed by hand has a higher fat content than milk expressed by pump (this is important to a mother who is expressing for a baby who cannot or will not feed).

The skin to hand contact helps stimulate your hormone responses.

It will teach you where the baby needs to be positioned on the breast to feed effectively.

If you develop any later problems like engorgement/mastitis then you know how to resolve it as it enables you to empty specific parts of the breast that may become blocked.

It is important to try and express your milk as soon as possible after your baby is born. To ensure that you produce plenty of milk, you will need to express at least six to eight times in 24hours, including during the night, just as your baby might be doing if they were able to feed directly.

Tip # 8:

If you feel your milk production is low go to your GP and ask for a medication called *'Domperidone'* it will increase your prolactin levels.

Chapter Four: Maternal Health and Well Being

Storing Breast Milk

You can store breast milk for:

Up to five days in the fridge at 4°C or lower. In order to achieve this it should be placed in the back of the fridge and not the door as this is the coolest part of the fridge.

Up to two weeks in the freezer compartment of the fridge

Up to six months in a domestic freezer compartment at minus 18°C or lower.

It should be thawed in a fridge and used straight away once defrosted. Never refreeze once thawed.

Correct positioning - I can't stress enough how important this is to get right in order to avoid complications. You have all probably read many books on this subject already but just a quick recap.

Baby to breast – always bring your baby up to the breast. Avoid bending/reaching down to meet your baby.

Nose to nipple – always ensure your baby's nose is opposite your nipple.

Back to back – always make sure that your baby is tilted over on their side so both your backs are in alignment. For more information visit http://www.unicef.org.uk

Avoid Use of Dummies

Dummies should be avoided in the early days. It is not entirely understood but is thought to be that the sucking motion of the dummy is different to that of the breast. With the breast, the baby draws the nipple back towards the soft palate at the back of the mouth whereas with the dummy the baby sucks with the hard palate towards the front of the mouth. Have you ever wondered why a breastfed baby keeps losing their dummy? This is the reasoning behind it. However, it has been shown that mothers who use a dummy are more likely to use supplementary feeds. The use of a dummy may mean that feeding cues are missed which may affect future milk production.

Avoid Supplementary Feeding

Each time your baby feeds, they are letting your body know how much milk to produce. The amount of milk you make will increase/decrease in line with your baby's needs. Breastfeeding works on a feedback mechanism. The more your baby feeds the more milk you will produce. If you introduce supplementary feeds this will upset nature's fine balance and much more likely to result in formula feeding your baby. Introducing infant formula will reduce the amount of breast milk you produce.

As a HV I know that not all mothers will breastfeed through choice or due to the fact that you may be returning to work or tried and not succeeded. While I know that breastfeeding is the best choice for babies I totally support all mothers who wish to use formula. The main thing is that mothers and babies are happy and healthy. Personally I feel it is unethical to judge any mother on her choice of feeding. Your decision should be respected as women are sometimes made to feel tremendous guilt about not breastfeeding and I think it is wrong. I know that women put enough pressure on themselves without professionals adding to it.

Chapter Four: Maternal Health and Well Being

Post-Natal Check and Exercises

Six weeks after having your baby your GP will offer you a post natal check. This used to be an internal examination but now it will only be a 'chat' like check-up, that is if you have had a normal straight forward delivery. If you have had a tear it is important that you heal fully and have no pain, especially after intercourse. Unfortunately, some women will have had a third degree tear which means that you will have torn all the way down to the anus or back passage. A fourth degree tear will involve the muscles of the pelvic floor, these women should have an examination at the hospital to ensure that there is no long term damage. In some cases a referral is needed to the physiotherapist to strengthen the muscles. In rare cases surgical repair may be required.

Many women will lose their sex drive after a baby, this is normal as you will be so tired from lack of sleep. Many women will not have had sex before their post natal check, whatever is right for you IS RIGHT. There are no hard and fast rules about when you should or shouldn't resume sex. I have had some women who have had sex straight after a baby and others who have not even thought about it until after the post natal check-up. But I do I get asked this question all the time by parents. What is important is that you feel physically and emotionally well enough to be intimate with your partner. You know when that will be.

I do advise carrying out some post natal exercises as this will help the pelvic floor muscles to get stronger. In pregnancy and birth the muscles become stretched and they need to tighten up again. This is important especially if you have had a long second stage-pushing, or multiple births. Many women regret not doing this when they spring a leak after a cough, sneeze or laugh.

Chapter Four: Maternal Health and Well Being

Tip # 9:

When passing urine try and stop the flow of urine halfway through by tightening your pelvic floor muscles. If you can stop the flow of urine – great; if not, get exercising NOW.

Contraception

You must, however, think about contraception as I have known women to be pregnant again at the six week check-up (my mother was one of them - sorry mum, she had 10mts between my older brother and sister). If you are breastfeeding on a regular basis you may not have a period for all the time you are breastfeeding. This is normal so don't panic if your level of 'prolactin' (the breastfeeding hormone) is high, this will keep your progesterone level low. Progesterone is the hormone that builds up the lining of your uterus in readiness for another pregnancy. Many women make the mistake of thinking they are not fertile if they are not having a period- WRONG. You will still be producing oestrogen and eggs will still be released. I am living proof of this, I was breastfeeding my first son exclusively for 10mts and I did not have a period in that time - (yippee!).

But I could not tell when I was fertile and I took a chance, had intercourse and ended up pregnant with my second son. Yes, I should have known better but even we professionals get it wrong sometimes. However, I didn't mind about being pregnant so quickly after my first baby so it did not matter to me. But if you do not want this to happen to you, you must use protection. Of course while you are breastfeeding you are limited about your choice of contraception as everything goes through the breast milk. You cannot take a combined oestrogen and progesterone pill while breastfeeding. The oestrogen will have side effects for your baby. You can take the 'mini pill' which is progesterone only. But you must be careful to take it at the same time everyday and if you have any vomiting or diarrhoea take extra precautions i.e. use condoms or you can get pregnant. Go and speak with your local sexual health clinic or GP as they will best advise you. In my opinion, it's best to keep it natural and use condoms until you have finished with breastfeeding your baby. But it is of course up to you.

Cervical Screening

A cervical screening test (previously known as a smear test) is a method of detecting abnormal cells on the cervix. The cervix is the entrance to the womb from the vagina. About 3,000 cases of cervical cancer are diagnosed each year in the UK, which amounts to 2% of all cancers diagnosed in women. In the UK every woman is offered a smear test every 3yrs between the ages of 25yrs and 64yrs.

Many women who are under the age of 25yrs old ask me that if they are sexually active and had a baby they should they have a smear test? I believe that the answer to this question is yes, but again it is a personal belief. As they, are more at risk of disease when sexually active, due to being infected with the HPV Human Papilloma Virus. This virus will make you more at risk, to prevent this virus girls of 12-13yrs are being offered this vaccination in school. However, GPs will not call you for a smear as you do not fit into the selection criteria. But if you go to a sexual health clinic they will rarely refuse you. It is however, uncommon but not unheard of to get cervical cancer under the age of 25yrs old. However, you may remember the case of 'Jade Goody' who died at the age of 27yrs old. She first had abnormal cells detected on the cervix at 15yrs old.

Chapter Four: Maternal Health and Well Being

If you are due a smear test, it is best wait to for 3mts after your baby's birth before having the procedure carried out. This is to allow the cervix to settle down after the birth.

Maternal Mood Assessment

Physical health of the mother is important but equally important is the emotional/psychological health of the mother.

Post natal depression is a major focus in the first year of the mother's and baby's lives and will be continuously assessed using the National Institute for Clinical Excellence (NICE) guidance. Screening should be carried out at regular intervals during the first year. Best practice is at the following times:

1. Antenatal visit
2. New birth visit (7-14 days)
3. Follow up visit (6-8 weeks)
4. 3-4 month review
5. 7-11month review

The HV will ask the following questions:

During the last month, have you often been bothered by:

- Feeling down, depressed or hopeless?
- Having little interest or pleasure in doing things?

Chapter Four: Maternal Health and Well Being

If a mother, answers 'YES' to these two questions and she accepts that she has feelings of depression and she would like to do something about her situation. Then the HV can proceed if trained and competent to carry out a further assessment by means of a screening tool known as the Edinburgh Post Natal Depression Score (EPDS).

Ideally this assessment should be carried out in the antenatal period as best practice. Many women become depressed in pregnancy and I believe it should be offered to every mother before the birth of their baby. Unfortunately, screening in the antenatal period is not common practice. It is for this reason I will be referring to women, as opposed to mothers.

This 10 item self-report (EPDS) measure is designed to screen women for symptoms of emotional distress during pregnancy and the post natal period. It is important to stress that the EPDS is not a diagnostic tool and must always be used in conjunction with clinical assessment. So if you have answered 'yes' to either of the above questions please go and seek medical advice and support from your GP, Midwife or HV.

The EPDS includes one question (item 10) about **suicidal thoughts** and is the most important to answer as honestly as you can. So you can get the correct support and help that you and your baby require.

The tool reflects the woman's experience in the last 7 days; the EPDS may need to be repeated on further occasions as warranted. If a woman answers 'yes' In HV practice this assessment tool should be carried out on three to four occasions; new birth visit, 6-8 week follow up visit, 3-4 month visit and again at the 8-11mt developmental assessment of your baby.

EDINBURGH POSTNATAL DEPRESSION SCALE (EPDS)

Question 1

I have been able to laugh and see the funny side of things:

As much as I always could

Not quite so much now

Definitely not so much now

Not at all

Question 2

I have looked forward with enjoyment to things:

As much as I ever did

Rather less that I used to

Definitely less than I used to

Hardly at all

Question 3

I have blamed myself unnecessarily when things went wrong:

Yes, most of the time

Yes, some of the time

Not very often

Hardly at all

Edinburgh Postnatal Depression Scale (EPDS)

Question 4

I have been anxious or worried for no good reason:

No, not at all

Hardly ever

Yes, sometimes

Yes, very often

Question 5

I have felt scared or panicky for no very good reason:

Yes, quite a lot

Yes, sometimes

No, not much

No, not at all

Question 6

Things have been getting on top of me:

Yes, most of the time I haven't been able to cope

Yes, sometimes I haven't been coping as well as usual

No, most of the time I have coped quite well

No, I have coped as well as ever

Question 7

I have been so unhappy that I have had difficulty in sleeping:

Edinburgh Postnatal Depression Scale (EPDS)

Yes, most of the time

Yes, sometimes

Not very often

No, not at all

Question 8

I have been sad or miserable:

Yes, most of the time

Yes, quite often

Not very often

No, not at all

Question 9

I have been so unhappy that I have been crying:

Yes, most of the time

Yes, quite often

Only occasionally

No, never

Question 10

The thought of harming myself has occurred to me:

Yes, quite often

Sometimes

Edinburgh Postnatal Depression Scale (EPDS)

Hardly ever

Never

It is important that you get help and support with your feelings. *If you have had any suicidal thoughts please go and see your GP today.* If you are just feeling low and want to talk to someone then contact your HV. If you can't get hold of her then come and speak with me, I hold support groups or one to one sessions as I am a qualified counsellor and coach (see back of book for details).

EDINBURGH POSTNATAL DEPRESSION SCALE SCORE SHEET

Question 1

I have been able to laugh and see the funny side of things:

0. As much as I always could

1. Not quite so much now

2. Definitely not so much now

3. Not at all

Question 2

 * I have looked forward with enjoyment to things:*

0. As much as I ever did

1. Rather less than I used to

2. Definitely less than I used to

3. Hardly at all

Edinburgh Postnatal Depression Scale (EPDS)

Question 3

I have blamed myself unnecessarily when things went wrong:

3. Yes, most of the time

2. Yes, some of the time

1. Not very often

0. Hardly at all

Question 4

I have been anxious or worried for no good reason:

0. No, not at all

1. Hardly ever

2. Yes, sometimes

3. Yes, very often

Question 5

I have felt scared or panicky for no very good reason:

3. Yes, quite a lot

2. Yes, sometimes

1. No, not much

0. No, not at all

Question 6

Things have been getting on top of me:

Edinburgh Postnatal Depression Scale (EPDS)

3. Yes, most of the time I haven't been able to cope

2. Yes, sometimes I haven't been coping as well as usual

1. No, most of the time I have coped quite well

0. No, I have coped as well as ever

Question 7

I have been so unhappy that I have had difficulty in sleeping:

3. Yes, most of the time

2. Yes, sometimes

1. Not very often

0. No, not at all

Question 8

I have been sad or miserable:

3. Yes, most of the time

2. Yes, quite often

1. Not very often

0. No, not at all

Question 9

I have been so unhappy that I have been crying:

3. Yes, most of the time

2. Yes, quite often

Edinburgh Postnatal Depression Scale (EPDS)

1. Only occasionally

0. No, never

Question 10

The thought of harming myself has occurred to me:

3. Yes, quite often

2. Sometimes

1. Hardly ever

0. Never

Please notice that questions 1, 2 and 4 are scored in sequence whereas all other questions are in reverse order.

Instructions:

Only score *one answer* in each section that is the most relevant and don't over analyse the question too much as this is your conscious mind talking. It is better to go with your 'gut/instinct' as this will be your unconscious mind speaking which always speaks the truth.

Try and be as honest as you can, nobody is going to judge you so you are safe. This is not an easy exercise to do but is so important for your emotional well-being.

Keep a running total and at the end of the 10 sections completed this will be your total EPDS score. Please see below for how to interpret the scores.

Edinburgh Postnatal Depression Scale (EPDS)

HOW TO INTERPRET THE SCORES

0-9: Scores in this range may indicate the presence of some symptoms of sadness/distress that may be short lived and are less likely to interfere with day to day ability to function at home or at work. However, if these symptoms have persisted for more than a week or two please go and talk to your midwife, HV or GP.

10-12: Scores within this range indicate presence of symptoms of distress that may be discomforting. Repeat the EPDS in 2 weeks' time and continue monitoring progress regularly. If the scores increase to above 12 assess further and consider referral as needed.

13+ Scores above 12 require further assessment and appropriate management as the likelihood of depression is high. Please go and see your GP as you may need some medication to help ease your symptoms. Depending on your score and your co-operation he may also suggest a referral to a professional in order to help you manage your anxiety and sadness for example - psychiatrist/psychologist/counsellor.

Your wishes should always be considered in this referral process.

If maternal mood assessment can't be carried out in the home (due to lack of resources) then it should be followed up when the mother attends the child health clinic.

Edinburgh Postnatal Depression Scale (EPDS)

NOTE:

Although postnatal depression is usually associated with new mothers, current research suggests that 1 in 25 new fathers are also affected.

Tips for Dads

- Talk about how you feel with family and friends.
- Allow time for yourself away from work and family.
- Try to maintain some hobbies or social events.
- Ask for help and support, you're not alone.

Chapter Five - Bottle Feeding

How to Recognise Signs of When Your Baby Wants to Feed

It is important that you recognise, when your baby is hungry as opposed to just wanting a cuddle, nappy change or sleep. Babies cry for many reasons and of course one of them is hunger. You will soon learn to recognise the different cries of your baby and the cry for hunger. But you should not have to let your baby cry to know when they are hunger. The signs of hunger in your baby can be picked up by the cues your baby gives you.

- When awake he will start to move about. This would be a good time to start preparing the feed.
- He will then begin to move his head and mouth around searching for food.
- Finally he will find something to suck, usually his fingers but it could well be your chin or nose whatever is handy. This is a good time to offer your baby his feed.
- If you miss these cues they will then start to cry.

Bottle Feeding

Infant formula is a minefield for most professionals to keep on top of let alone new parents as there are now so many different formulas and different types of milk within each brand. It is impossible to keep up with technology and marketing. There seems to be different milks to respond to every different need, it can be very confusing.

Chapter Five – Bottle Feeding

Most infant formulas are made up of the same nutritional content based on skimmed cow's milk and is treated so babies can digest it. Vegetable oils, vitamins, minerals and fatty acids are added to make sure the milk contains the vitamins and minerals that young babies need.

Breastfeeding is the preferred method of feeding and should be promoted by all health professionals. If, however, a mother is unable to breastfeed, or after discussions about the benefits of breast-feeding chooses to bottle feed, I believe you should be supported in your decision by all health care staff. Parents should receive adequate advice about:

- Infant formula
- Food preparation
- Sterilisation of equipment

It is recommended that, if an infant is not breastfed, formula should be continued until the age of one year as it is higher in iron than cow's milk. Babies must never be left alone with a bottle, especially overnight as this can lead to:

- Choking
- Increased risk of dental caries

All formula should be made up according to the manufacturer's instructions. The following are examples that should not be added to bottle:

- Sugar
- Honey
- Cereals including Rusks, Cerelac, and Raab.
- Milk flavouring products or other solids

This practice may:

1. Block the teat
2. Lead to choking
3. Result in dental caries
4. Lead to poor nutrition and Obesity.

Water can be offered between feeds. Fruit juice is not necessary and can cause erosion of the tooth enamel with frequent use. If given after 6 months old, it should be well diluted and, preferably, given only at mealtimes.

Addition of Nutrients to Formula

No artificial feed can completely mimic the nutritional and protective properties of breast milk. Manufacturers of some infant formula milk in recent years have supplemented them to be as close to breast milk as possible.

All cow's milk based formulas are suitable for vegetarians as they no longer contain beef fat. All infant formula sold in the UK must meet the guidelines set out in 'Artificial Feeds for the Young Infant'.

Types of Milk

Infant formula is produced from modified cow's milk. There are two types; these are whey dominant and casein dominant formulas. The infant formula and follow-on formula regulations regulate minimum and maximum nutrient concentrations and the food ingredients that can be used in the manufacture of infant formula.

Standard Infant Formula

Whey dominant formula (commonly called first milks) has 60% Whey: 40% Casein ratio. They are closer in composition to breast milk than casein dominant formula and have a lower renal solute load.

Examples of whey dominant formulas:

- Formula Manufacturer
- Aptamil -Milupa
- First Milk Farley's
- Infant Milk formula 1 Boot's
- Cow & Gate - Premium Cow & Gate
- Gold SMA
- Sainsbury's First Stage Milk

Casein dominant formula (commonly called second stage milks) has 20% Whey: 80% Casein ratio. Casein forms curd, which are thought to be more slowly digested, and these milks are promoted as being more satisfying for hungry babies. There is currently no scientific or medical evidence to support this thinking. Furthermore, there is no evidence that casein dominant formulas lead to a later introduction of solids as has been suggested. It is better to choose one milk formula and stay with this without making changes. However, some mothers may choose to change formula because the baby is experiencing problems like vomiting or regurgitating. There is no evidence that this is necessary or beneficial.

Examples of casein dominant formulas are:

- Formula Manufacturer
- Milumil -Milupa
- Second Milk Farley's
- Infant milk Formula 2 Boots

- Cow & Gate Plus Cow & Gate
- White SMA
- Sainsbury's Second Stage

If a mother chooses to bottle feed their baby, whey dominant formula should be the first choice for newborn babies, and can be continued throughout the first year of life.

Vitamin D Supplements

Vitamin D is very important for you and your baby. It helps your bodies to absorb calcium, which is essential for keeping bones healthy throughout life. Vitamin D helps to make sure that babies' bones and teeth remain strong. It is recommended that all babies from six months should be supplemented with vitamin D drops especially if taking less 500mls of formula per day. Breastfed babies should be supplemented from one month if the mother has not taken vitamin D supplements during pregnancy.

Low levels of Vitamin D in babies and children can lead to rickets, which affects the way bones develop and grow. The bones of a child with rickets are unable to support their weight, resulting in bowed legs and knock knees.

Signs and Symptoms of Low Levels

Bone and muscle pain

A soft skull

Weak teeth and delayed growth of teeth

Delayed walking

In severe cases it can result in low calcium levels in the blood – leading to muscle cramps, seizures and breathing difficulties

Case Study

I had a mother who had experienced a difficult c-section birth, the baby was pulled out by his leg. This led to her baby having a hairline fracture of his thigh bone (undetected at birth). Within weeks he accidentally had a fall from his crib and sustained a fracture of his skull. This made the doctors in A&E suspicious. The baby had a full skeletal survey carried out and the previous leg fracture was picked up. The family were accused of non accidental injury of their baby and he was placed on the child protection register. This family's life was turned upside down. They were treated like suspects and had 2years of social workers in their lives. The baby had a low Vitamin D level which led to the fractures.

Follow-on Formula

Follow-on formula contains higher levels of certain nutrients compared with breast milk or standard formulas:

Protein

Iron

Vitamin A

Vitamin D

Follow-on formula is not suitable as a replacement for breast or formula milk for infants under six months because of its higher protein and other nutrients which can put the kidneys under added stress

Chapter Five – Bottle Feeding

when digesting. Follow-on milks are not essential and it is perfectly acceptable for a bottle fed baby to continue on ordinary infant formulas after 6 months. Although they contain more iron and vitamin D than ordinary formulas, it is not known how much of this iron is readily absorbed. There is no evidence that they offer any advantage over an adequate mixed diet containing sufficient iron-containing foods plus whey or casein based formula.

Examples of Follow-on Milks Are:

- Follow-on
- Formula
- Manufacturer
- Follow-on Milk Boots
- Follow-on Milk Farley's
- Forward Milupa
- Progress SMA
- Step - up Cow & Gate
- Follow-on Hip Organic

Cow's Milk

It is strongly recommended that cow's milk is not introduced as the main milk drink until the baby is 1 year of age, as cow's milk is an inadequate source of iron and contains high solute load. It also provides added vitamin content compared to cow's milk.

However, it can be used in small amounts to mix solids from 6 months of age (see more on this under weaning). Cow's milk given to young children must be pasteurised and stored in a fridge. If unmodified cow's milk is introduced at age 1 year, it should be full fat or homogenised until the child is 2 years of age. Skimmed and semi skimmed milks have a lower energy and fat-soluble vitamin content than full-fat milk and are not suitable for children under the age of 2 years. Semi-skimmed milk can be given to children from the age of 2 years and skimmed milk from the age of 5 years.

Condensed milk, evaporated milk, sheep's milk and goat's milk, or any other type of drinks (such as rice, oat or almond drinks, other known as 'milks' should not be given to a baby under one. You should not use soya milk unless it has been prescribed by a doctor. Evaporated and condensed milks are not suitable for infants as they contain high sugar content. Foods made with cow's milk such as custard and milk puddings, and other dairy products such as cheese and yoghurt, may be introduced in small amounts at any time between 6 months and 1 year. It may be advisable to delay the introduction of dairy products for longer in babies with a family history of atopic disease.

Goat's and Sheep's milk

Goat or sheep's milk should not be given to infants under 2 years of age. Goat's milk is low in folic acid and vitamin B12. Sheep's milk is far higher in protein, fat, energy and minerals and is the least similar to breast milk. Older children having these milks need additional sources of folic acid and vitamin B12 from iron-rich foods or as a supplement. Although goats and sheep's milk may be perceived as being less allergenic, or providing special nourishment, none of these claims have been substantiated. Both contain lactose and therefore offer no benefits for infants with lactose related diarrhoea. Advice from a dietician should be sought. Unless the parents feel strongly about giving these milks, they should not be recommended. These milks may not be pasteurised and so need to be boiled before giving to young children. Vitacare Ltd has produced a modified goat's milk formula called Nanny. This guideline does not recommend the use of NANNY for infant feeding, as it is manufactured from modified goat's milk and this does not comply with the Infant feeding and Follow-on Formula Guidelines (1995). It is also unsuitable for older infants /children with milk intolerance as the protein composition is very similar to that of cow's milk and the chance of cross reactivity is high.

Soya Infant Formulas

Specialised formulas are for infants with special medical requirements. Infants may have medical conditions where a special diet is indicated and/or may require specialised formula milk or a supervised feeding plan. These formulas are available on prescription. Any infant/ child who is on a specialised formula should be under the care of a Paediatric Dietician.

Babies under 6 months of age who do not tolerate cow's milk formula or are at high a risk of allergy should have an extensively hydrolysed formula such as:

Formula Manufacturer

Nutramigen- Mead

Johnson

Pepti Junior- Cow & Gate

Pregestimil- Cow & Gate

Soya based infant formula should be prescribed by a Paediatrician, GP or Dietitian and only where clinically indicated.

Examples of Soya infant formulas, which meet the Guidelines for the composition of infant formula, are:

Soya Formula Manufacturer

Infasoy - Cow & Gate

Isomil - Abbot Nutrition

Farley's - Soya

SMA- Wysoy

Prosobee- Mead Johnson

Cow's Milk Protein Allergy (CMPA)

CMPA is difficult to diagnose as the signs and symptoms are so wide and varied. It can manifest as a number of different signs and symptoms, mainly affecting the skin, gastrointestinal tract and the respiratory tract. There is no official guidance on the diagnosis of this allergy but should be considered if there is a family history of allergy. Or where there is any of the following symptoms like; babies/children who suffer from moderate to severe or eczema, gastro-oesophageal reflux disease or other gastro-intestinal symptoms including, colic, loose stools and constipation that have not responded to the usual treatments or interventions.

Personal Story

When I was on holiday with my first son he had just turned four months and back then the advice was to wean onto solids at that age. I started him on some baby rice and mixed it with some formula milk. I had not given him either before as he was fully breastfed. He hated the spoon and the taste but I persevered despite my baby trying to tell me (by pushing the food out with his tongue) that he did not either want the spoon feed nor like it, I persevered as I really wanted to enjoy my holiday and hopefully get him sleeping through the night. Having battled through my first attempt at weaning I decided that it was not a great success.

We all went out shortly after the feed and my poor baby spent the remainder of the evening being sick. The following day I decided to give him some formula to see if it was the baby rice that had upset him. I soon discovered that it was the milk as he again vomited up the formula milk. He was irritable and unsettled for the following few days. I decided not to give him any more formula. When we returned home from holiday I tried again to introduce solid food by giving him just fruits and vegetables which he was fine with. At 5mts I tried again introducing cereal to him with breast milk but again he was sick and then his weight started to drop. I decided to ask for a referral to a specialist as I thought there might be an underlying problem.

It turned out that he had both cow's milk and wheat allergy.

Skin symptoms include:

Immediate signs:

- Itching
- Redness of the skin
- Urticaria/hives large well defined swellings (most commonly on the lips and face and around the eyes)

Delayed signs:

- Above first two signs
- Eczema

Gastro-intestinal system symptoms include:

Immediate signs:

- Swelling of the lips, tongue and palate
- Mouth itching

Chapter Five – Bottle Feeding

- Nausea and vomiting
- Diarrhoea
- Colicky abdominal pain

Delayed signs:

- Gastro-oesophageal reflux disease
- Loose or frequent stools
- Blood and or mucus in stools
- Abdominal pain
- Infantile colic
- Food refusal or aversion
- Constipation
- Redness around the anus
- Pallor or tiredness
- Failure to thrive or gain weight

Respiratory System symptoms include:

- Upper respiratory tract symptoms- nasal itching, sneezing, runny nose/discharge
- Lower respiratory tract systems – cough, chest tightness, wheezing or shortness of breath

Other signs include:

Sudden onset of difficulty in breathing may include swelling around the lips and mouth – otherwise known as anaphylaxis. This will need urgent attention.

NOTE: The only definitive diagnosis for CMPA is allergy testing that is how my son was picked up. (Ask at your GP or you can go private).

Chapter Five – Bottle Feeding

Pre-term Babies

There are a number of formulas available in the UK, which are designed specifically for the low birth weight /pre term baby. These formulas have a higher nutrient density than standard formulas and contain adequate nutrients for most pre term babies, although, some may require additional iron and vitamin supplements. If a pre-term infant is unable to tolerate cow's milk based formula, they should be referred to a Paediatric Dietician for further advice. Soya based formula are not recommended. GP's are now able to prescribe Nutriprem2 and Premcare until 6 months of age. Pre- term babies can sometimes be challenging to feed as they tire easily.

How do I Encourage my Baby to Feed Correctly From a Bottle?

- Always hold your baby close to you when you feed and look into their eyes when feeding. This makes your baby feel safe and loved. Never prop feed a baby or leave them alone with a bottle as it is a choking risk.
- Try to hold your baby upright, with the head supported in a comfortable neutral position.
- Brush the teat against his lips and when he opens his mouth wide with his tongue down, help him draw the teat in.
- Hold the bottle horizontal to the ground, tilting it just enough to ensure that your baby is taking in milk, not air, through the teat. Babies feed in bursts of sucking with short pauses to rest. In this position, when your baby pauses for a rest the milk will stop flowing, allowing him to have a short rest before starting to suck again.
- You will see bubbles in the bottle as your baby feeds. If you can't see any bubbles, break the suction between his tongue

and the teat from time to time by moving the teat slightly away from him to the side of the mouth. You should then see bubbles rushing back up into the remaining milk.
- Your baby may need to burp so allow him to have short breaks during the feed, the amount of breaks will vary on the age and amount of feed for each baby but most babies will only require one or two breaks.
- Interrupting the feed from time to time with breaks will also allow your baby a chance to register how full he is and whether he needs to complete the full feed. Don't make him finish the bottle if he doesn't want it.

Bottles and Teats

Bottles should be made from a hard plastic with the opening big enough to make them easy to clean. There are many manufactures that claim their teat is similar to the shape of breast, that is sadly not the case as teats cannot lengthen like the human breast/nipple. Teats can be made from rubber or silicone and vary in shape, there are some that are labelled orthodontic teats which follow the line of the palate and some mothers feel that these are easier for their baby to feed from than the simple long teats. There is no evidence that one teat is better than another, babies are all different and you will just have to experiment and find the one that is right for your baby.

However, what is important is the size of the hole in the teat. As a guide when you turn the bottle upside down the milk should drip out as a rate of one drop per second. Your baby should be able to complete their feed within a 20min period. If they are taking much longer than this they will tire and give up on the feed. This is especially the case in preterm babies where their sucking is weaker.

Chapter Five – Bottle Feeding

You can choose the flow of the teat to suit your baby's needs they will vary depending on the manufacturer from one hole in the teat (slow flow) to four holes (fast flow). If the milk is flowing too fast for your baby they may drool in order to protect the airway. In this instance it is of course better to change to a slower teat. The flow of the teat will have an impact on the amount of wind your baby will accumulate.

Wind

Most babies swallow air when feeding which may lead to wind. This can occur in both bottle-fed and breast-fed babies. Winding the baby once during the feed and afterwards for about five minutes should be enough. Persistent winding can upset the baby and cause vomiting.

If your baby shows signs of distress during a feed, encourage them to let go of the teat and sit them up to burp. Continue to feed them when they are more comfortable.

Causes of Wind in Breast-Fed Babies

The infant is incorrectly positioned at the breast and has not "latched on" properly or does not feed long enough at one breast (see chapter on breast-feeding).

Causes of Wind in Bottle-Fed Babies

The hole in the teat may be too small. The milk should fall in a constant run of droplets when the bottle is inverted. A slow feeder may benefit from a larger hole and a hungry fast feeder from a smaller one. The bottle may not be tilted enough and the teat traps air instead of being full of milk. To get rid of this the teat should be moved to the side of the mouth to allow air to enter the mouth and to get rid of the vacuum.

Your baby should take about 20mins to feed try not to hurry a feed. However, if your baby is taking longer than 30mins then you need to get a faster flowing teat as they will get exhausted from sucking. Prolonged crying, which causes the baby to swallow air, this also is a cause of wind.

How Often Should I Feed my Baby?

In the early days and up to 6-8 weeks health professionals will recommend that you feed on demand. Therefore you should feed a baby as much as she wants, or as often as she asks, provided she is not regurgitating significant amounts. If she is regurgitating significant amounts this may be a sign that they want smaller amounts but possible more often than want is recommended on the tin guide.

Newborn babies will take quite small amounts to start with, but by the end of the first week of life most babies will ask for about 150-200mls per kg per day (see next chapter on frequently asked questions – question 2 for an example of how to work this out for your baby) although all babies are different and this amount will vary from baby to baby until they are six months old.

Chapter Five – Bottle Feeding

Tip # 10:

Try to avoid giving too much milk or using the hungrier baby milk in the hope that your baby will go longer between feeds. It is just going to create problems with your baby being sick, gaining too much weight or having digestion problems like colic.

Colic

The true definition of colic is a baby who cries for 3hrs on three consecutive days for three weeks. A baby who cries for shorter periods or intermittently would not be a baby who has colic. It is often called "evening", "infantile" or "three month colic". It may begin soon after birth and continue throughout the first few months. The cause is unclear but the signs and symptoms are abdominal distension or bloating of the tummy, pain, flatulence and long bouts of crying. The baby screams and pulls up the arms and legs, nothing seems to comfort the infant for more than a few minutes. It is important to exclude other factors like cold, hunger and poor feeding technique.

Management

The baby normally appears healthy and thriving; although very distressing for both you as parents and your baby, it is self-limiting and will gradually resolve itself. There are certain techniques that will help ease the pain. Holding the baby prone across the knee or regular massage of the baby's abdomen may give comfort. Cooled boiled water may help. A drink of diluted herbal tea such as fennel, camomile, balm mint or liquorice seems to be an effective treatment but not definitely established. Mothers of breast-fed babies can drink the herbal tea. A change of feed is not helpful and may aggravate the symptoms. There are agencies out there that will help like 'Cry-sis', a voluntary group that will give a listening ear and practical advice.

Drug Treatment

Over-the-counter colic drops like' Infacol'(brand name) may help to improve the symptom; it is non-toxic and not absorbed. It is said to act by altering the surface tension of mucous, allowing entrapped gas bubbles to join together and be more easily released by the mouth or anus. The other colic drops available are called 'Dentinox' (brand name) which has the same ingredient as Infacol. Sometimes I think that these drops are more effective for the parents in that you feel you are doing something to ease your baby's discomfort.

There is now another preparation on the market called 'Colief' but is only useful for pain associated with lactose intolerance.

If you do have any issues around feeding your baby it is important to attend the baby clinics to have your baby weighed and to have any of your questions answered by the health visitor. The next chapter will cover what happens in the clinic visits. Clinics are there as a resource for you to use but many parents do not attend or take u the free advice that is on offer. This may be the only opportunity to see a HV; especially if you live in an area where you only see your HV on a single occasion (new birth visit) due to low resources.

Chapter Six- Health Education and Promotion

Clinic Visits

Clinic visits are not just for monitoring your baby's growth, it is an opportunity for you as a parent to talk about how you are feeling. Yes of course, it is important to go and see your HV at regular intervals to ensure that your baby is growing normally along their birth percentile. Percentile means that if you take one hundred babies, fifty percent of the babies out of that one hundred will fall on the 50th percentile or otherwise will be of average weight.

Clinic visits are important for your baby as it is the only concrete way that you as the parent will know if your baby is thriving and getting enough milk/nutrition to grow. At birth your baby will be weighed and his/her weight will be plotted in the red book.

Percentile/Growth Charts

The growth charts are found at the back of the red book and will be identified as graphs. You will notice that they include the following:

0.4th percentile

2nd percentile

9th percentile

25th percentile

50th percentile (average)

Chapter Six – Health Education and Promotion

75th percentile

91st percentile

98th percentile

99.6th percentile

Your baby will be born on one of the above percentiles at birth and should remain on that percentile for normal healthy growth. All babies are different in size and it is not useful to compare your baby with others but it is natural. These differences will be down to parent's size and the culture into which that child is born. For example Asian babies tend to be smaller than average and Afro-Caribbean babies tend to be bigger than average. When you visit the baby clinic your baby will be weighed and plotted every time you attend. This will be by a member of the support staff. If there is any deviation from normal you will be advised to see and talk with a HV.

How to Interpret the Graph

As mentioned previously, the percentile charts are based on a measurement out of one hundred children. Fifty percent of the population will fall on the 50th percentile and if that is the case for your baby they will be within *'average'* of the total population.

NOTE: No baby is average in my opinion they are all unique and special. This is for illustration purposes.

If your baby is on the 75th percentile they will be above average and if they are on the 25th percentile they will be below average. It is important to say that it does not matter on which percentile you child is born whether, they are bigger or smaller is not a reflection on how healthy they are. What is important, however, is that where they are

Chapter Six – Health Education and Promotion

born they remain, they should not deviate too much from their birth percentile unless there is a minor issue.

There are of course times when this does happen. If your baby is unwell, with sickness or diarrhoea for example, they will lose weight. This is to be expected and normally when better the weight will improve and return to normal. Sometimes your baby may be unwell with an underlying infection for example, ear/throat/chest infection and again they will lose weight. But the weight should return to normal when your baby has recovered from their illness. However, if your baby is losing weight with no explanation then this is more cause for concern. Babies who lose weight without any reason should be monitored and kept close watch on as it can be an early sign of some underlying health concern. If there is no improvement in the weight within four weeks and your baby continues to lose weight then medical help should be sought by seeing your GP.

On the other hand if your baby gains too much weight this is also a matter of concern. Babies who are obese in childhood are more prone to ill health as adults.

For an example of both boys and girls growth charts please see overleaf. It is important that your baby's given the right growth charts as the boys chart will be slightly different from the girls chart. Boys grow at slightly faster rates than girls. If you look closely at the charts you will see the differences.

NOTE: Most babies will grow along their birth centile. If they deviate up or down by one centile don't worry. If they deviate by two centiles, we will simply monitor the situation and may refer to the GP for opinion.

(Growth Charts on next page taken from Parent-Held Record/Red book)

Chapter Six – Health Education and Promotion

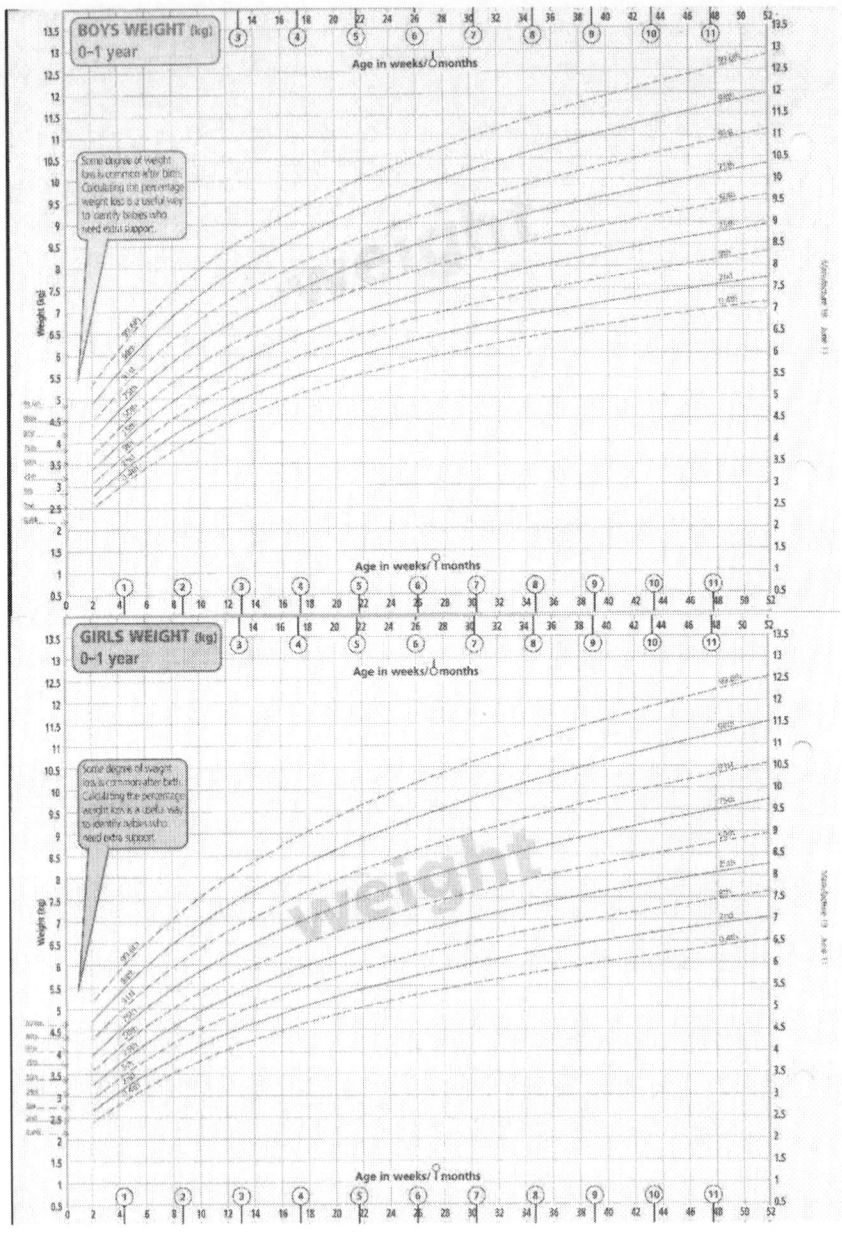

Chapter Six – Health Education and Promotion

Top 10 Questions Asked of Health Visitors

Clinic visits are the ideal opportunity to ask your HV about any questions you may have about your baby. I have been asked hundreds of questions over my 20yrs as a HV on every aspect of parenting here are the top 10.

Question 1

My baby is breastfed. How do I know my baby is getting enough milk?

Your baby should be content and gaining weight.

In the first 48 hours, your baby is likely to have only two or three wet nappies. After this they should become more frequent in number up to six every 24 hours from day five onwards.

Most babies lose up to ten per cent of their birth weight and this is acceptable. From day five to seven they should have regained their birth weight.

Your baby's first stool (poo) is black in colour and known as 'meconium'. By day three it should be changing to lighter, runnier, greenish stool. From day four your baby should pass about two soft, yellow stools per day, a bit like mustard in texture. Many breastfed babies will pass many more in number and these can be quite runny which is totally normal. However, I have known some breastfed babies to also go without passing a stool for up to a week and then have an 'explosion'. Please don't worry too much as long as your baby is feeding and not being sick then he/she does not need intervention. They have simply used up everything they need and no waste. I see many new mothers running off to A&E with their newborns thinking they are constipated (I will cover this in detail in a later chapter. Then, babies being given suppositories (little capsules placed into the anus) to 'make them' open their bowels.

Question 2

How much weight should my baby put on each week?

Table 1

Age in months	Weight gain per week in grams
2 weeks - 4 weeks	200g (6 oz)
4-8 weeks	150g (5 oz)
8-12 weeks	90g (3 oz)

NOTE: 30grams = 1 oz (ounce) 16 oz =1 lb (pound) and 14lbs = stone.

To calculate the expected weight of an infant:

The following information is needed:

1. Age of baby in weeks

2. Birth weight

3. Knowledge of expected weight gain (See Table 1)

4. Knowledge that baby will not regain birth weight until age 10 to 14 days.

Chapter Six – Health Education and Promotion

Example

Infants age   8 weeks

Birth weight   3,400 g (3.4 kg)   7lb 8oz

200g (6oz) gain/week

For (8-2) weeks – as baby will take 2 weeks to regain birth weight (but not always)

= 200g X 6 weeks = 1,200g   1,200 (1.2kg)   2lb 10oz

Or 7oz X 6 = 42oz

Therefore the expected weight = 4,600g (4.6kg)   10lb2oz at 8 weeks

Question 3

My baby is bottle feeding. How much should I feed by baby?

Your baby will require 150mls of formula milk per kilo of body weight, divided by how many feeds per day. So if we take the example above:

150(mls) X 4.6(kg) = 690mls in 24 hrs this would normally be 5 bottles

$$\frac{}{5} = 140\text{mls or roughly 5oz (30mls =1oz) per feed}$$

If your baby was feeding 3hrly then the above figure would be:

$$\frac{150 \times 4.6}{8} = \frac{690\text{mls}}{86\text{mls or roughly 3oz 3hrly}}$$

It is important not to over feed your baby as it may lead to the following problems:

Your baby being overweight leading to obesity

Digestion problems –'possetting'/regurgitation, vomiting, constipation

Question 4

My baby won't settle and he keeps bringing milk up. What is wrong?

Once you know how much your baby should have in volume to grow normally then it is important not to give them any more than their body needs to digest. Many parents will over feed their baby in order to pacify them and stop them crying. Babies love to suck, it soothes them and the sucking reflex is very strong in the first few months of life. If you give your baby a feed and it is not due a feed they will suck to soothe themselves. By doing this they obviously take in milk and this can cause them to bring milk back.

If it is only small amounts this is normal and is called 'possetting' (this is NOT vomiting) health professionals will often call it 'regurgitation'. Sometimes your baby will do this naturally when being winded.

If your baby has just had a feed or had one less than an hour ago they should not be hungry. However, it is important to say that your baby may be thirsty especially in hot weather. The foremilk will quench thirst. The hindmilk will satisfy hunger (more on this in later chapter). If your baby has too much foremilk this can sometimes result in 'green poos' being passed.

Chapter Six – Health Education and Promotion

They may be unsettled for other reasons: tired, bored, wanting a cuddle. It normally takes a baby at least an hour to digest food but can take up to two hours. If you try and feed a baby when their stomach is still full this will result in the baby being sick or vomiting back the feed. If the baby has a partly full stomach then this will have started to curdle from the hydrochloric acid –this is the first stage of the digestion process. If fresh milk is put down on top of this partly digested milk it can also make the baby feel sick.

Chapter Six – Health Education and Promotion

Question 5

Why does my baby look smaller/bigger than other babies the same age?

When your baby is born their weight will be plotted on their birth percentile chart, these are the charts/graphs at the back of your baby's 'red book'. If you go to your red book, you will see that the pink chart is for a girl and blue for a boy. It is important that they are charted correctly as boys and girls grow at slightly different rates. Babies will vary in size depending on factors like ethnicity and family make up. Usually 'smaller' mums will have smaller babies but not always. For example, some cultures, like Afro Caribbean tend to have bigger babies than white Caucasian and Asian babies tend to be smaller.

The main thing that your Health Visitor (HV) will be looking for when you come to clinic with your baby is that your baby is following along on their birth percentile. So if your baby was born on the fiftieth percentile (50th) that means that out of one hundred babies your baby is of average size. If they are on the twenty fifth (25th) percentile they are below average and if on the seventy fifth (75th) percentile they are above average size. But it is important to stress that whether they are above or below it doesn't make them better or worse, just different. It is best that your baby follows their birth percentile. That means they are getting enough nutrition to grow and develop at a normal pace. If your baby deviates from this there is normally a reason i.e. they may have had a cold and not feeding well or they could have had a 'tummy bug' and will lose some weight. They will normally make it up within a few weeks. If they have not been ill it is best to see the HV to have a talk about feeding to see if there are any underlying problems that need addressing.

Chapter Six – Health Education and Promotion

Question 6

I am worried as my baby's stool is 'green' in colour and sometimes it is 'seedy' in texture. Is this normal?

Many breastfed babies have stools that are 'seedy' in texture. This is completely normal and nothing to worry about. It can also be a result of something the mother has eaten.

It is more common for bottle fed babies to have green stools but some breastfed babies can also have 'green' stools. The reason behind this is that formula milk has got many additives to make it as near to breast milk as possible. However, the iron that is added to formula milk is sometimes not needed by the baby, so the baby's body will get rid of it by passing it through the digestive system. This will make the stool turn green.

Sometimes mothers who are breastfeeding will be on extra iron supplements due to a bleed in delivery or just low iron levels and she will require additional iron tablets to correct the anaemia. If your baby does not need the extra iron, again it will simply be passed through into the stool. In either case this is nothing to worry about. Your baby will remain well and healthy.

In rare occasions, babies do pick up bacterial or viral infections and this will make your baby feel unwell. If your baby develops a high temperature, is unsettled and crying or stops feeding then you will need to see a GP.

Question 7

My baby is vomiting every feed and won't keep his milk down. What should I do?

I have already spoken about how to define regurgitation, now let me define vomiting. Vomiting - is a reflex action and common in childhood. If the stomach is bloated (over full) or irritated it will reject its contents. Vomiting is when your baby brings up sufficient milk that it will make a puddle on the floor or soak his clothes through. It is ok for your baby to vomit from time to time. But if your baby is vomiting up most of the feed on each feed there is a problem and you need to see a GP.

There are many reasons why babies vomit from the minor to the more serious:

- Overfeeding
- Not being winded properly or sufficiently
- Reflux
- Infections
- Milk allergy
- Milk intolerance

Underlying medical condition i.e. hiatus hernia (a condition in which part of the stomach protrudes upwards into the chest through a hiatus or opening normally only for the oesophagus in the diaphragm), pyloric stenosis (narrowing of the outlet or pylorus of the stomach that obstructs the passage of food into the bowel).

I have already mentioned about how to avoid over feeding. Make sure that you wind your baby frequently during a feed.

Some babies need more frequent winding than others. How much wind your baby will accumulate will depend on the type of bottle and teat that you use.

Chapter Six – Health Education and Promotion

Mild Reflux

Reflux is a condition where the contents of the stomach come up the food pipe or oesophagus in small but frequent bouts. Some babies will experience reflux as a newborn. This is due to the muscle which keeps the stomach contents down being over-relaxed. This is made worse if the baby is particularly active or of handled too much after a feed. The muscle will strength will increase as the baby gets older.

TIP: Always place your baby in a head up position after having a feed and avoid laying them straight down as this will help minimise the problem. Place a rolled up towel or pillow under the top end of the mattress at night. NEVER place a baby directly on a pillow as this is dangerous. Always place the baby feet to foot of the crib/cot.

More Severe Reflux

If the baby does not lose weight then mild reflux is simply a nuisance in having to wash baby clothes more. But if your baby is losing weight because of the amount he/she is bringing up then this will need intervention. See your HV who will advise you on treatment. The first line is a special milk which is a 'thickened formula' which will help if bottle feeding. Each brand will do their own, for example, SMA call it 'stay down' milk and Aptamil call it 'anti reflux'. If your baby is breastfed then go and see your GP who will prescribe medication that will help. Gaviscon is the usual medication of choice but if this doesn't work then there are others. This does tend to make your baby a little constipated. Ranitidine or domperdone can also be prescribed.

If your baby is allergic to 'cows' milk protein' then they will have an adverse reaction to formula milk. This could be vomiting or it may be other gastro-intestinal symptoms like diarrhoea. It is important to have this diagnosed by a GP and get the correct treatment.

Chapter Six – Health Education and Promotion

Another reason why babies vomit is from intolerance, for example 'lactose', it is important that your baby gets the correct diagnosis and then the correct treatment will follow. Don't be afraid to ask your GP for a referral to a specialist doctor.

In rare occasions your baby could possibly have an underlying medical problem. So always seek help if none of the above is apparent. If your baby continues to vomit they quickly become dehydrated.

Question 8

How do I recognise if my baby is dehydrated?

Babies will have several signs if they are dehydrated and it needs to be corrected as soon as possible or your baby is at risk of harm.

Signs and Symptoms:

- Decreased urinary output
- Dry nappies
- Dry skin, lips and mucus membrane (inside their mouth)
- Sunken eyes
- Sunken fontanelle (soft spot on the top of your baby's head)
- Lethargy (your baby may sleep more than usual)
- High temperature - May lead to convulsions (fits)

If your baby has more than three of these signs; or if your baby is refusing fluid of any kind then go and see your GP. If concerned go straight to the hospital. Avoid the milk as it may be making the problem worse. Go to a chemist and get rehydration solutions i.e. Dioralyte. This will replace the lost fluids and correct the imbalance which will make your baby feel better. Check your baby's temperature (normal temperature between 36.1 and 37.2 degree celsius) by using a digital thermometer try and reduce it by cooling the environment for

Chapter Six – Health Education and Promotion

example - take clothes off, open a window, tepid sponge (luke warm water) your baby and allow the droplets to evaporate which will have a cooling affect. If your baby is old enough (minimum 8 weeks) then give Calpol (infant paracetamol) 2.5mls only.

Infection

High temperatures can also be caused by infections. Signs of infection are reduced feeding, irritability and lethargy. If a baby's temperature remains high you should go and see your doctor. Your baby should not go longer than 24hrs if they have a fever as they may have an infection.

Many babies get infections, the most usual are:

- Gastroenteritis (Diarrhoea and Vomiting)
- Otitis media (ear infection)
- Tonsillitis (Infection of the tonsils)
- Chest Infection
- Bronchiolitis (Infection of the small airways in the lungs)

Question 9

My baby has colic. What should I do?

Colic is crying for 3hrs for 3 consecutive nights for a period of 3 weeks. It is associated with excessive air swallowing or faulty feeding formula or technique. It is recognised by the frequent, intermittent bending of the legs and can be associated with back extension. The tummy will be distended (bloated). Trapped wind causes pain and must be released. If a baby is unable to do this for themselves then they will need assistance.

Prevention is the best policy:

Check that you have the correct attachment of baby to breast. Could possibly be a problem with positioning?

Check that there is no presence of tongue-tie problems.

Check you are making up feeds correctly with the cool boiled water before adding the formula.

Try not to overuse Cool boiled water as supplement to feeding.

Use the correct teat flow size for your baby (1-4 holes in teats).If your baby is taking in too much air they are more at risk.

Ensure frequent winding throughout the feed.

Make sure your baby does not get too hungry as they are more likely to gulp in air.

Treatments will vary but those most frequently used are – Infacol, dentinox and colief (the latter is mainly used for pain associated with lactose intolerance rather than colic).

Both bottle and breastfed babies can suffer from colic. It is most prevalent in the first 3mts of life and does improve with the introduction of solid food.

Question 10

My baby is 4weeks old and hungry all the time. Can I give my baby the hungrier milk formula?

First formula milks are designed for newborn babies as the protein in them is made up of 'Whey'. This protein is easier to digest and goes through the digestive tract quicker than the step 2 milks for hungrier babies.

Chapter Six – Health Education and Promotion

Many babies will stay on the first step formula milk all the way up to a year old. The difference between this formula and the step two milk; is in the protein - 'casein'. This harder to digest and sits in the stomach for longer and forms a curd which goes through the gastro-intestinal tract more slowly. For this reason many parents choose it, to get longer periods between feeding.

The difficulty is that, the younger the baby is the harder they have to work to digest the 'casein' which puts strain on the gut. This may lead to many problems like constipation and colic. Many babies are not ready for this hard to digest protein and experience 'gut ache/colic' in trying to digest something that their body is not ready for. The gut then has to work so much harder resulting in all the water being drained off and this leads to hard painful stools. I am going to speak about constipation as a separate issue as it is so common.

Other Minor Problems

What is Constipation?

Many mothers' feel that their baby is constipated if they don't have their bowels opened daily. They become concerned and will phone me up for advice, if their baby has not had their bowels opened for 3 or 4 days. I always reassure them that this is not a problem as long as when your baby opens their bowels the stool is soft. It is not unusual for a baby to go up to a week without passing a stool, especially if they are breastfed. If your baby is tolerating feeds and showing no signs of distress try not to panic.

Constipation is when the babies' poo' is dry, hard, infrequent and it looks like rabbit pellets in appearance. To avoid constipation occurring check that feeds are made up correctly and the amount of feed given is right for your baby. The first line of treatment is to increase fluid intake by offering cooled boiled water between bottle feeds. If this doesn't work, then, and only if your baby is over 6mts of age (ideally) you can give well- diluted (at least 1:12) unsweetened fruit juice – prune, apple or pear (if water is not accepted). Its use should preferably be limited to after feeds.

The use of sugar or honey in water is not recommended. Once, the baby is taking solids, unsweetened fruit or vegetable purees may help. Babies over 6 months may be given more fibre-rich foods e.g. Weetabix, wholemeal bread, beans and lentils. Never give raw, unprocessed bran. If none of this works then a referral to GP is recommended if there is no improvement. Laxatives (stool softeners should not be given unless recommended by a medical practitioner).

Breastfed Babies

Just because your baby does not 'poo' everyday does not mean your baby is constipated, it should not be defined solely as the infrequent passage of stools. True constipation occurs when the stool is hard and difficult to pass. There is a great variation on how often stool is normally passed and it will differ with each individual baby, but further investigation should be considered if longer than 5 days has elapsed since the last motion. Constipation is unusual in the exclusively breastfed baby, although infrequent stools, once every 4-5 days, are not uncommon but even with delays exceeding this the stool should be the soft/loose stool typical of the breastfed baby.

Bottle-Fed Babies

Inadequate fluid/over concentrated feeds – check that feeds are being made to the correct dilution and that the water is measured in the bottle before adding formula. If the feed is being made up correctly, increase fluid intake by offering cooled boiled water between feeds. If water is not accepted, well-diluted unsweetened fruit juice may be offered, after 4 weeks of age.

Underfeeding – check the amount of feed given per kg of expected body weight in 24 hours and increase if necessary. Organic obstruction is rare, but should not be forgotten in breast or bottle fed babies, especially when there is vomiting and/or abdominal distension. Urgent investigation is needed if the vomit is bile (yellow) stained or projectile (forced out and goes across the room).

In hot weather, particularly, extra water may be needed for bottle-fed babies. Over- clothed babies in over-heated homes should be made cooler by removing the extra clothes and decreasing room temperature. The use of sugar or honey in water should not be used. Once the baby is taking solids, unsweetened fruit or vegetable purees may help.

In older babies (6+ months), the consumption of other fibre-containing foods can be increased, i.e. wholegrain cereals, beans and lentils, remembering to offer drinks frequently.

Older Children

Constipation may occur at the time of toilet training. An adequate fluid intake should first be ensured; 1200-1500ml/day, depending on the child's age, is recommended. In children over 2 years, dietary fibre can be increased gradually. Suitable fluids include water, milk and well-diluted fruit juice. Tea, coffee and other drinks containing caffeine, such as cocoa and cola drinks, have a diuretic effect (which makes the child urinate more frequently and hence loose fluid more quickly) and should be avoided. Excessive milk intake, that reduces the child's appetite for more fibre-containing foods, should be restricted to the recommended volume for that age. Good sources of fibre include wholemeal bread, wholegrain cereals,(e.g. Weetabix, Shredded Wheat and porridge), beans, lentils, fruit and vegetables (especially peas and sweetcorn). The child should be encouraged to establish a regular bowel habit and rewarded with plenty of encouragement and praise.

What is Diarrhoea?

Diarrhoea is the frequent passage of stools and where the contents of the stool is fluid like and seeps into the nappy. If it last longer than 24hrs your baby will be at risk of dehydration.

Medical advice must be sought if dehydration is suspected. The use of oral rehydration (diorlyte sachets) solutions is recommended for the prevention of dehydration during diarrhoea and for the treatment of mild dehydration. Breastfed babies should continue breastfeeding during rehydration.

Bottle-fed infants should be given only oral rehydration solutions for the first 24 hours, unless symptoms are very mild. They must not be kept solely on oral rehydration solutions for long periods. Solids should not be given for at least 24 hours, but prolonged periods without food are inappropriate. Give a dry diet and avoid anything dairy (over 6mts) as this will aggravate the bowel.

Babies

It is important to establish what the normal stool pattern is and to identify any innocent causes of diarrhoea such as a change in diet. It may take several days for a baby's stool pattern to settle down after the introduction of new foods. Diarrhoea may be caused by an infection, feeding too concentrated infant formula, sugary drinks or an allergic reaction.

Dehydration

Dehydration is a common and a potentially serious problem, occurring in many illnesses of babies and young children, particularly gastroenteritis. It is caused either by inadequate fluid intake or excessive fluid losses due to fever, sweating, vomiting and/or diarrhoea. Mild dehydration is difficult to detect. Therefore, if suspected, medical advice must be sought. Established signs including thirst, lethargy, irritability, loss of skin elasticity, dryness of the mucous membranes, reduced urine flow, fast heart rate, fast breathing and sunken fontanelle indicates significant dehydration and the need for urgent medical attention.

Prevention and Treatment of Dehydration

The use of oral rehydration solutions, for example during episodes of diarrhoea, is an effective way of both preventing and treating mild dehydration. Suitable solutions include; dioralyte or rehydrate. Follow the manufacturer's instructions as to their use. An adequate volume of fluid should be given initially every hour, or more frequently if vomiting occurs. Fluid intake should keep pace with any losses.

Breastfed babies should continue to be breastfed. Bottle-fed babies should be given only oral rehydration solutions for the first 24 hours, unless symptoms are very mild. Oral rehydration solutions contribute insignificant quantities of nutrients, other than water and electrolytes, and bottle-fed babies must not be kept on these alone for long periods. Oral rehydration should continue, in addition to appropriate nutrition, until the diarrhoea stops. There is no good evidence to suggest that diluted feeds are preferable to full strength feeds after rehydration. Special infant formulas are rarely indicated.

Medical referral is recommended if vomiting, fever, or blood in the stool accompany diarrhoea. Children under 5 should be excluded from nursery or other early years care until they have had no diarrhoea or vomiting for at least 24 (and preferably 48) hours.

Older Children

Toddler diarrhoea is a common problem in children who are otherwise healthy. The child has increased stool frequency and undigested, recognisable foods such peas and carrots are seen in the stools. The child remains well and normal weight gain continues. Toddler diarrhoea is a harmless condition. The diarrhoea may be helped by reducing fibre intake (e.g. changing to white bread instead of wholemeal and choosing a refined breakfast cereal such as Cornflakes or Rice Krispies). Many toddlers have a high intake of fruit juice and squash that they drink purely for the flavour. It is better to reduce the amount of concentrate and increase the amount of water; this will help reduce the number of loose stools per day in toddler diarrhoea. The condition often improves spontaneously at around 3-4 years of age

Chapter Seven – You and Your Baby's First Year

In chapter I outlined the new birth visit and what to expect. For many mothers this may be the first and last time that you will see your HV, this is a common occurrence as at the time of going to print there is still an ongoing shortage of HVs and you may feel alone in your parenting and unsupported. You may only see a HV in the baby clinic setting, that's if you choose to attend. For those of you who are lucky enough to be in an area where staffing is not an issue you will be visited at home on more than one occasion.

1. New birth Visit (7-14 days)/Maternal Mood Assessment
2. Follow up visit (6-8 weeks)/Maternal Mood assessment
3. Weaning visit (3-4mts)/Maternal Mood Assessment
4. Developmental Assessment (7-11mts)-usually invited to clinic/Maternal Mood Assessment

I will therefore focus in more detail on the content of these visits within this chapter for those of you who may not be offered a visit or don't get the opportunity to ask your own HV at clinic. At each of these visits it is an opportunity for your HV to re-assess your mood to screen for post natal depression.

Chapter Seven – You and Your Baby's First Year

Follow up Home Visit by Health Visitor (6-8 weeks)

The follow up visit is important as usually at this time the husband/partner has gone back to work. All visitors and family members will be gone and the mother will be coping alone. By now there should be some sort of routine established for the mother and baby.

Baby

The baby should have had the BCG (only offered in high risk areas) carried out by this visit and the first developmental check should have been booked at the GP surgery. Feeding should be less demanding and baby should be getting into a routine. You should have been to your baby clinic and had your baby weighed at least once if not twice. I say SHOULD but not always.

Mother

You as the mother should be recovered from the birth experience. The breastfeeding should be well established and you should be feeling more like your old self. You should have by now booked your post natal check with the GP.

The HV will look in your baby's red book to see how your baby's weight is progressing. She will ask you about the feeding and how it is going or if you are experiencing any problems. She will answer any questions you may have.

The HV will talk about your health and well being if you are eating and drinking well. She will assess you for any signs of post natal depression. Many women who have felt happy up until now may be experiencing some stress now that you are on your own and having to do

Chapter Seven – You and Your Baby's First Year

everything. You will feel tired from broken sleep and may now be feeling a little low in mood. That's OK, just talk about your feelings and let your HV or GP know how you are feeling.

First Developmental Check 6-8 weeks

As outlined in the first section of this book the 6-8 week developmental check is the only check that is not carried out by the HV. This is a physical check of your baby is the only check that is carried out by your GP. (All other developmental checks are carried out by your HV). This is a crucial check to have carried out and I cannot stress enough how important it is that you attend with your baby.

It will basically be a repetition of the newborn baby check that your baby had carried out in the hospital. The focus is on four main areas:

Eyes

Your GP should carry out a routine inspection of your baby's eyes looking to see if they are focussing and moving their eyes. The GP is looking for any signs of cloudiness which could indicate a problem known as newborn cataract. This is rare, only about two or three babies out of 10,000 will have a problem. They should carry out a more thorough examination of the eye with an ophthalmoscope to check the back of the eye.

Heart

The GP should listen to your baby's heart with a stethoscope they will be listening out for the normal noises made by the heart. Sometimes heart murmurs are picked up and this can be worrying for you the parent. Some babies are born with heart murmurs and they cause no health problems whatsoever. There will not require any intervention at all, it just means that there is an extra noise made by blood as it passes through the heart. If the GP picks up anything that is concerning he/she will refer you on to a specialist for their opinion. Around one in 200 babies have a heart problem that will need treatment.

Hips

It is important if your baby is born breech (bottom first) that they have their hips closely examined as these babies are more prone to hip problems. All babies born in this way will be offered an ultrasound of the hips to check the stability of the joint. Some baby's who present head first can also have hip problems and if left untreated can lead to joint problems and possible limp. If the GP is concerned, again he/she will refer you to a specialist for treatment. Only one to two babies out of a 1,000 will be born with hip problems.

Testicles (not checked in all areas)

All baby boys will be checked to see if the testicles are able to be brought down into the scrotum. It can take several months for the testes to come down and in rare cases this may not happen. They will be checked again at health review by age one (7-11mt check) as different areas do it at different times. If they are not down by age one to two years then the GP will refer your baby to a specialist for a minor operation to bring them down. About one in a 100 baby boys will need treatment.

Why Attend this Developmental Check?

This check is the most important check of your baby's life in my opinion for all the above reasons. I have seen a baby at 6 weeks who was invited by the HV service for a routine 6-8 week developmental check to be carried out by their GP. I, the HV present at the clinic that day carried out his height and weight check prior to the physical check being carried out. Therefore, I was able to see this baby naked prior to his check with the GP. This is now not normal practice, most babies are weighed by support staff and not seen by a HV unless you specifically request it. This is fine if you just want your baby weighed but if you want advice please ask to see a HV.

Case Study

When I saw this baby I could tell straight away that he was very ill. He looked frail and when weighed had not put on any weight. He also looked thin, he was blue around the lips and having difficulty in breathing (nasal flaring and laboured breathing). I had a suspicion that he had a significant heart condition. (I had worked on the cardio-thoracic unit for children with heart lung defects at Great Ormond Street Hospital).

Baby A had the newborn check carried out at the hospital and nothing of note picked up. He did not come to the baby clinic for any weight checks until his invitation for the 6 week developmental review. He had lost weight and weighed less than his birth weight. He had difficulty in feeding as he was so breathless he couldn't suck. This baby was rushed to hospital. He had a major heart condition and needed urgent medication and surgery to save his life.

I don't know why this baby's heart condition was not picked up at the antenatal screening. It is possible that the mother did not attend the ultrasound scans. I also don't know why the doctor did not pick up the defect when this baby was born at his newborn baby check. He may have been a junior with insufficient experience. He may have been tired or even have taken a shortcut or he could simply have forgotten. I know that young doctors work too many hours and that is not an excuse but a possible explanation. I don't know the answer. But I do know that if this baby did not attend for his 6 week developmental check on that day it is a real possibility that he may have died.

After this review you should attend the clinic for regular weighing to ensure your baby is thriving, as you may not see your HV again at home for a long time, if ever. If you are lucky you may get a home visit to discuss weaning onto solids at home.

3-4 month Home Visit (Not All Families Will be Offered This Visit)

Weaning onto Solids

This visit is an opportunity to carry out more health education and promotion. This is an opportunity to advise and guide you the mother about weaning onto solids. In the first six months of life breast milk or infant formula provides all the nourishment your baby needs. Weaning is not recommended under 17 weeks of age at the earliest, your baby should ideally be able to do the following before commencing solid food;

Sit up without support. It is safer and easier to feed your baby once they are sitting.

Pick up foods and put them in their month.

Chew food- babies do not need to have teeth to chew.

Swallow rather than suck. They use their tongue to move food from front to back of mouth.

Chapter Seven – You and Your Baby's First Year

It is important not to reduce the amount of milk your baby is having until your baby is fully weaned i.e. having three meals a day. Getting your baby used to eating solid foods is more important than how much they eat. However, at first your baby will still need more breast milk or infant formula than solid food. Only when they start eating more solid food should you reduce the amount of milk they are having.

Cutting Down on Milk Feeds

Once they are on three full meals a day then you can reduce the milk down, it is important that they have a minimum of 500mls per day = 16 ounces. This is to allow them to have enough calcium for their teeth and bones. If your baby does not have this amount then you can give them other calcium sources like cheese or yogurt. You can start giving babies cows' milk in your cooking or when mixing their food from six months. However, if they are having a drink of milk, it is important not to give cows' milk until after 1 year old. After this time the milk can be reduced to 300mls or half a pint of full fat milk. If they drink too much milk this will fill them up and they will not be hungry enough for food.

Chapter Seven – You and Your Baby's First Year

Hints:

Home- made foods are cheaper, better tasting and help prevent your baby from being a fussy eater later on. Make a big batch of fresh vegetables, fruits, stews or savoury pies (like shepherds or cottage pie). Freeze the food in containers, then you will just have to defrost them as needed.

Encourage finger foods straight away, this is called 'baby led weaning'. Babies enjoy finger foods and it helps build confidence to self feed as well as encouraging hand eye co-ordination and fine motor development.

It's good to give your baby a wide range of healthy foods early on. It doesn't matter which foods they try first, but make sure you offer a variety of foods.

You baby will let you know when they are full. They will turn their face away, close their mouth or push the food out with their tongue.

Remember your baby will need to learn how to eat solid foods. If they don't seem to want the foods you offer, try them again on another day. It takes about 15 tries before your baby develops a taste for new foods.

All babies are different. Be patient in getting your baby used to new foods.

I find that a combination of both these methods is the best approach. But you as parents will have your own preferred approach. Just ensure that you offer a balanced diet from all food groups. As long as your baby is gaining weight that is the main thing.

Chapter Seven – You and Your Baby's First Year

Foods to Avoid

- Salt and Salty foods- avoid adding salt to your cooking. Processed foods are higher in salt and should be avoided. Gravies and stock cubes are also high in salt.
- Sugar and sugary foods- Do not add sugar to foods, it will make your baby develop a sweet tooth and more prone to weight gain.
- High fibre foods- too much fibre can prevent the absorption of iron. Introduce slowly and don't overload their system.
- Foods low in fat- babies need energy to grow but they will get this from full fat dairy products.
- Honey should not be given under a year old as occasionally it can contain bacteria (botulism) that can make your baby seriously ill.
- Whole nuts and grapes are a choking risk. Crush nuts and cut grapes to avoid the risk.
- Under cooked eggs, meat and fish. These should all be fully cooked.

Gag Reflux

A gag reflex is nature's way of moving food from the back of the throat into the front of the mouth. Learning to move food this way is how your baby learns to chew and swallow food safely. Gagging is noisy and when a baby gags, they may turn red in the face, but they will usually continue to eat. It is when your baby is not making any noise, this is when you need to take fast action.

I recommend all new parents to take a first aid course.

Dental Hygiene

Your baby will get teeth any time between birth, (yes some babies are born with teeth) and one year of age, but the majority will be around six months of age. Whatever the age it is important that when they do get teeth that you start to brush them with a small soft toothbrush and only a smear of family fluoride toothpaste. Many parents will over fluoridate and this can lead to white marks being left on the teeth. Your baby does not need baby toothpaste as long as you DO NOT put too much toothpaste on the brush; a smear of toothpaste is sufficient (1000ppm up to 3yrs of age and 1350-1500ppm thereafter, pea size). Too much fluoride can cause white spots on the teeth. Most areas will fluoridate the water and some areas add more so check out your areas policy.

Drinks

Milk and water (cool boiled rather than bottled) are best for teeth. From six months a free flowing cup can be introduced. By one year infants should have all drinks from a cup and the bottle should be weaned off to prevent any malformation of the teeth. Sweetened tea, juices and sugary drinks will lead to tooth decay if taken through a bottle. These drinks are best avoided or kept to a cup if given. It is best to give water or milk.

This will be the last visit to take place at home and many will not be offered a home visit to discuss weaning. You can always speak about this in clinic if you are unsure and need guidance.

Returning to Work

Many mothers are thinking about returning to work at this time and it is still possible to continue to breast feed your baby, if you should wish to. Many women will feed before and after work which is sufficient milk for your baby as long as they are on solid food. If you can express and give the bottle to the nursery/child-minder this is the ideal, but if you can't then your baby will be fine with a formula feed. If your baby refuses formula don't worry as long as your baby is taking water from a cup they will not become dehydrated. Your baby only needs 600ms of milk for healthy teeth and bones you can supplement with other calcium sources like cheese and yogurt, as long as your baby is six months old.

Childcare

Returning to work is difficult for any mother, but don't feel guilty if you are looking forward to going back to work we are all different in our needs. Many women choose to take a full year off work but many will have to return once their pay reduces to the statutory maternity benefit. Some mothers' may not be entitled to any maternity allowances, for instance if you are self-employed or on a zero contract.

Childcare is one of the biggest concerns for parents returning to work. It is important to consider your options and there are pros and cons for all:

- Family
- Childminder
- Nursery
- Nanny
- Au-pair
- Share it between you and your partner

Family

If you are lucky enough to have parents living near you and they are in a position to help with childcare, then this is the ideal option. As you will be save thousands of pounds and know your baby will be loved and safe.

Child-minder

If you want your baby to be in a home environment then this is the option for you. Child-minders will also offer you much more flexibility with their hours, in that, they may be willing to start earlier and finish later. They may also be able to assist with babysitting or even an overnight stay. However, if the child-minder is sick, on holiday, they may not be able to take your child. Some child-minders operate a 'buddy system' to allow for these eventualities. In these circumstances your baby will go to the buddy child-minder.

The downside for some mothers is that there will be other children and these may be older or even school age children, so your baby will be out and about for school runs. If you and your baby, are happy with this then this may be a cheaper option to nursery or nanny. All child-minders now have to offer your child the early years' foundation stage curriculum so they should be having structured play sessions. You need to ask what they can offer your child and look for evidence. They are also inspected by OFSTED so you can look them up on the website.

Nursery

Childcare is very expensive and on average most nurseries will charge you about one thousand pounds per month for a full time place (2014). The advantages are that your baby will be looked after with children of their own age (this may be a disadvantage for some) and there will be no issues around holiday or sickness so pretty much guaranteed childcare. Again, if your child is sick, the same rule applies. They will not be permitted into the nursery. The times will be fixed usually 8am until 6pm and if you are late you will pay a hefty late fee. All nurseries are vetted by OFSTED every 3 years, but will also have a local authority inspection every year.

Nanny

If you want your baby to remain in your home and have guaranteed flexible childcare then this is the option for you. This is the most expensive option for childcare but, along with the childcare the nanny will carry out light household and all the care associated with your baby, like washing and ironing of baby's clothes. This has to be negotiated into their contract, you may also want to include babysitting or overnight stays. It's pretty much a contract between you and your employee as they are primarily self-employed. In addition to paying a salary, some will also request that you pay their tax and insurance. Nannies are not vetted by OFTSED and are pretty much independent. Unless, they have come to you via an agency, then the agency will carry out all the checks as part of the service.

Au-Pairs

Au-Pairs are a cheaper alternative and they can come from anywhere in the world, primarily to learn English and experience the culture. They will live full time with your family, so you must have a spare room. They will do house cleaning, washing/ironing as well as child care duties in exchange for room and meals. It can be quite intrusive to your family, having a stranger come into your house. The rules have recently changed on Au-Pairs and now they can no longer be in sole charge of a baby under 2yrs. So if you have older children, this may work well. There are two options with childcare you can go for basic package which means that they will work a couple of hours in the morning and then another couple of hours in the evening. You can also request an extended package Au-Pair Plus where they work full time for you. Most will want the first option, as their main objective is to learn English, so they will want to attend ESOL (English as a second language) classes along with time off to discover the sights. It may work for some families more suited to older school age children.

Share Between You and Your Partner

This can be very tiring and rewarding, for both of you and of course will only work if you work shift hours. I know many nurses, police officers etc to work in this way. Some will choose to use a combination of family, nursery and parents but it can be hard to juggle and a bit confusing for everyone to manage, so you need to be well organised.

You must find what is right for you. Please do give it some thought once you become pregnant and don't leave it until the last minute. I see so many parents in a panic about childcare when it is time to go back to work. You need to be securing a nursery place sometimes a year in advance, in order to get a baby place. Nannies and child-minders also get booked up months in advance so be prepared especially if you have no family around to support you.

Chapter Eight - Sleep and Behaviour

It is not recommended to train your baby to sleep under the age of six months. The ideal opportunity to speak about sleep training is at the 7-11mt developmental check. This is a good time to approach the subject only if it is a problem for the parents. Some parents don't mind getting up in the night to feed or comfort their baby. However, by now your baby should be sleeping on their own, in their own room. But of course it is your decision.

Why is Sleep so Important?

Sleep is so important for both you and your baby, if you don't get enough sleep you will become unwell, either in body or in mind. Sleep deprivation is a form of torture and is very effective at wearing you down both physically and emotionally. It is by far the biggest problem I get asked about as a HV.

The Impact of Sleep Deprivation on Children

- Obesity-hormone influence
- Learning problems
- Accidents
- Hurtful behaviour
- Hyperactivity-ADHD (Attention Deficit Hyperactivity Disorder)
- Decreased IQ levels
- Behaviour problems

Chapter Eight – Sleep and Behaviour

The Impact of Sleep Deprivation on Parents

- Irritability/short temper
- Tension
- Lack of concentration
- Confusion
- Headaches
- Mistakes at work/home
- Weepiness/crying
- Anxiety/depression
- Chronic fatigue and tiredness
- Ill health-physically or emotionally
- Aggression

What is a Sleep Problem?

The following examples are typical of sleep problems:

- Need the breast or bottle to get them to sleep
- Babies over six months or young children who still wake for a feed during the night
- Need to be rocked to sleep
- Need a parent in the bed to fall asleep
- Can only sleep in their parent's bed
- Can only fall asleep on the sofa
- Refuse to go to bed
- Refuse to stay in bed
- Wake during the night
- Wake early in the morning

Chapter Eight – Sleep and Behaviour

Advantages of a Good Sleep Pattern

- Improved behaviour in the child
- Greater harmony within the family
- Less parental anxiety
- Improved functioning at home and work
- Boosts the immune system
- Improves the psychological and physical development of the child
- Improves cognitive function

How to Teach Your Child to Sleep

There are two main methods of teaching your child to sleep, I personally do not recommend sleep training until your baby is at least six months old. The reason being is that by now you should have started solid food and thus your baby should not be waking for hunger. They also may now be in their own room.

The first method is called gradual retreat; If your baby is refusing fluid of any kind

The best way to avoid sleep problems is to prevent them happening in the first instance.

<u>Step One</u>:

Every baby should be put down to sleep awake. Your baby needs to learn how to go to sleep on their own without the breast, bottle or you

Chapter Eight – Sleep and Behaviour

for comfort. If you use any of these as a means of getting your baby to sleep then you are teaching them bad habits. You are teaching them to associate going to sleep with a comforter. So by all means feed your baby before a sleep and give them a comforter/transitional object to replace you (a soft toy or blanket). Make sure to put them down when semi awake so they know they are going in their cot. Many parents make the mistake of cuddling, rocking or soothing a baby to sleep.

Step Two:

Your baby should be able to go to sleep within 15/20 minutes of being put down to sleep. If not then you need to look at factors that may be affecting this from not happening. For example, is the time you are settling your child off to sleep right? What time was their last nap? Was it too near to bed time? Is there a bedtime routine and is it consistent?

Step Three:

Keep nap times regular and consistent. As a rule of thumb if your baby is under a year old they will need two naps a day, one in the morning lasting about an hour and another one around lunchtime for about an hour. Try to avoid late afternoon or early evening naps. After a year old your baby should have reduced down to one nap per day around lunchtime for an hour to two hours. By two or three years your child will no longer need naps.

Step Four:

In order for your baby to sleep you will need to keep the room quite, dark and a comfortable temperature. Always sleep your baby in the room in which they will be sleeping at night for consistency. Avoid letting your baby sleep in the car, pram or sofa as it breaks the consistency. Sometimes of course this is unavoidable. If you can implement these four steps it will reduce sleeping problems from occurring.

Method One - Gradual Retreat

This method is based on the concept of parents slowly distancing themselves from their child. It is a lengthy process that can take many weeks to achieve. You will start the process by sitting beside your baby's cot with your back slightly away from your child so there is no eye contact being made. You are physically present but emotionally absent from your baby (some parents find this difficult). Some parents start by holding their baby's/child's hand through the bar of the cot, others start from lying beside their child. It depends on how you have taught your child to sleep as to what will need to be undone or re-learned. Obviously this level of contact will take much longer to break.

You then gradually take a step further away each night until you are out of the room and your child is going off to sleep on their own.

This method is suitable for:

- All ages from babies to teens
- Building confidence
- Anxiety issues related to sleep and separation
- Parents who want a gentle/slow approach
- Room sharing siblings

Method Two – Controlled Crying

Controlled crying is a shorter and quicker approach but is not for the faint hearted (as you will see in my case study below) and can be tough on the parent emotionally. It involves placing your child in the cot awake and leaving the room totally. Then at brief intervals returning to check your baby's safety and to reassure your baby that you are still there. The timing between visits is up to the parent to set for themselves as some parents can handle longer spells than others and I would not want to dictate on this. Anything from 5mins to 20mins is usual depending on your comfort level; I usually recommend starting with 5mins and working up to 20mins intervals.

When you go in to check your baby, just look through them if you can, try not to make eye contact. You are carrying out safety checks to ensure that your child has not got caught up in bedcovers or been sick etc. If all is well with baby then just leave the room. It is important not to talk to your baby or pick them up which is difficult, especially if they are distressed and holding their arms out to you. You can place them down in the cot and 'tuck them in' but do it with haste and intent. If you are going to say anything it should be with a firm and determined tone 'IT'S TIME TO SLEEP'. It will be hard but you must be consistent in your approach. It is no good going in and speaking softly and gentle to your baby. You will be rewarding the undesired behaviour and you will confuse your child. Be assertive in both your tone and body movements, this will give your child a firm message that you mean business. Keep checking until your baby goes off to sleep. You need to repeat this procedure every time your child wakes in the night which can be exhausting but don't give in or give up.

IT DOES WORK, I promise. This is what one of my mothers' said:

Chapter Eight – Sleep and Behaviour

Testimonial

"Ann, I wanted to say a huge thank you for the advice you gave me with our son last week. He has slept through the night for the first time in 14 months. I can't believe it was so easy to do".

It does not come this easy for everyone though, I found it much harder.

Personal Story

When my first son was 10mts old he was still waking in the night for a breastfeed. I was a softie and continued to feed him although I knew he wasn't hungry as he was fully weaned onto solids, he simply liked the comfort. I became pregnant again at this stage (another story) and I was very tired as I also had just returned back to work after a year off. I knew I had to take some action to deal with the disrupted sleep as I was exhausted. I used to run a sleep clinic before I went on maternity leave so I knew the theory but my emotions prevented me from implementing the theory.

I decided to take action and implemented the controlled crying method. I chose to start at a weekend as my husband would be home and he could help me and give me strength if I was 'wimping out'. So we started on a Friday evening, I put Ben to sleep as usual at 8pm following his bedtime routine of bath story and breastfeed. The first half of the night was fine as he usually didn't wake until about 1-2am. The first night we went to Ben 35 times I couldn't bear to leave him too long and 5min intervals was all I could cope with emotionally in the beginning but slowly increased it to 10mins and then 15mins. It was 4am before he finally settled after three hours of on/off crying. My heart was breaking. Everything inside of me as a mother wanted to reach out to him and comfort him, but I stayed strong emotionally.

The second night he woke three times and settled within half an hour of crying. By the third night he was sleeping through. I could not believe it took only three nights to solve this problem although it was really tough on me and my husband we had succeeded as we were consistent and never gave in to his crying. It had paid off, he was sleeping through after that and we never looked back.

Tip # 11:

Remember be consistent and think, ask yourself am I rewarding 'good' or 'bad' behaviour? If you pick your baby up, you are rewarding the undesired behaviour and it **will** continue. It is up to you the parent; you are in control.

Older Child Who Repeatedly Gets Out of Bed

Version of controlled crying for a bed sleeping child

A stair gate across the bedroom door creates a room sized 'cot'

Child proof the room before starting

Use at bedtime and repeat each time your child wakes up

Nightmares

Nightmares occur during the second half of the night, during REM- rapid eye movement sleep or active sleep. Your child will wake and be crying, anxious and afraid for some time, they will find it difficult to settle back to sleep as they often still remember the pictures or content of what the nightmare was about. When your child wakes they will be distressed and will remember the experience in the morning.

Chapter Eight – Sleep and Behaviour

Hints for Parents:

- Ensure bedroom is not scary for children- avoid pictures or soft toys that can cast shadows
- Give attention immediately and comfort until the child is calm
- Give your child an opportunity to talk about the dream at the time if right, or in the morning
- Always try and settle them back in their own bed rather than yours to prevent a sleep problem occurring
- Try and turn the nightmare into a happy ending to enable your child to settle back to sleep
- Explore if your child is currently experiencing any fears/anxieties at home or school
- Avoid any scary movies or books before bedtimes

Night Terrors

These can start before the age of one but are most common in three and four year olds. Usually the child will be heard screaming and thrashing about but they are still asleep. They tend to happen after the child has been asleep for a couple of hours and are in non REM sleep or deep sleep. When you enter the room they will sit bolt upright and look terrified but they have no recollection of the event in the morning. Your child will normally grow out of them. You should not wake your child during a night terror, but if you notice a pattern of them occurring at the same time each night. It may help to wake your child about 15mins beforehand. Keep them awake for a short while, about 5mins, this should be sufficient time to break the cycle, then allow them to settle back to sleep. This will help to prevent it from happening again. Although distressing to watch they are not dangerous for your child.

There are triggers that can set off a nightmare and often if a child is sleep deprived this will exacerbate the frequency of occurrence. Some stimulates will also trigger the nightmare like caffeine or excess sugar can contribute to them. To avoid it happening it is important to have regular naps and set bedtimes which establish body clock thus reducing the occurrence. They can run in families.

Behaviour Issues

When you see your health visitor for the 2-2.5 year developmental check your child's behaviour will be discussed.

There is a strong link between behaviour issues and lack of sleep. However, many young children simply go through tears and tantrums in their twos and threes. One of the many reasons is that they are exhausted or feeling overwhelmed with life. There is a developmental reason for this; toddlers are very ego centric at this age, this means that everything is about them. You will hear them say 'me', 'mine' and 'I want' and if they don't get want they want they will act out or have a tantrum. Typical issues they will be presenting with are:

- Being bossy
- Being fussy
- Being clingy
- Being fearful

Temper Tantrums

Temper tantrums are a way of toddlers being able to express their confusing and strong feelings. Sometimes they can't express how they are feeling in words and when it all gets too much they simply have to release all those feelings. They are not doing it, just to get attention; it is a coping strategy for them. Some of these feelings are tiredness, anger, fear, frustration and rage to name but a few. They can be difficult for the child to cope with and they need to know that they are loved despite these strong feelings being displayed. It is important that you can show them that you still love them despite their behaviour. Even when your child is out of control you as the parent must stay in control of your own feelings and manage your own state which can be challenging at times.

Try These Helpful Hints:

Try counting to 10 before you take any action but make sure that your child is safe first.

Distraction can be useful if you can see the tantrum coming or escalating.

Avoid times and places when you know they are more likely to occur (sweet shops or supermarket) and have a plan in mind (bring some grapes/bread sticks with you).

Don't ask more of your child than they can handle as they can become overwhelmed very easily.

Try not to get drawn into an argument with them about what started it as they probably can't even remember and are past caring.

Try to avoid, for example saying or doing things that will hurt them back, especially threats of leaving them in the supermarket or having them 'taken away' as I have heard some parents say. You know you don't mean it but they don't.

Don't worry about them growing up to be a monster. They will grow out of them slowly but it may take time.

Remember that this is how they are learning to manage their feelings and learning lessons about themselves. (It is good practise for when they become teenagers believe me, I've got three of them).

Sibling Rivalry

Toddler tantrums often coincide with the arrival of another baby. The arrival of a new baby is often a very difficult time for the older sibling and of course they have been used to getting all the attention up until now. They did not choose to have the baby, you did and this can cause lots of new feelings that your toddler may not have experienced before. There can be intense feelings of jealousy and fear of being 'pushed out' with the arrival of a new baby and anger towards both the baby and the parents. This can be challenging to deal with when you are tired and lacking in sleep as you have limited resources to deal with these issues.

It is important to prepare your child for the new arrival. I am often asked by parents: when is a good time for to plan a second baby? My thoughts on this are personal and what is right for me and my family would not necessarily be right for you and your family. All I can say it that I had an 18mt gap between my first and second child and experienced no sibling rivalry. I then had a 3yr gap between my subsequent children and again no sibling rivalry. I may have just been lucky as none of my children really had toddler tantrums either. I consider myself lucky rather than anything to do with my parenting.

I have seen lots of different reactions from siblings in my 20 years as a practising HV. Here are some of those reactions:

1. Some children quite clearly try to physically hurt their baby when they arrive or openly say they don't want them and to give them back.

Chapter Eight – Sleep and Behaviour

2. Others are very loving towards their baby, but aggressive and angry to the mother.

3. Some become very withdrawn and show regression in their behaviour in order to get the mother's attention, for example, bedwetting in a previously dry child or ask for a nappy to be put on. Some will want to breastfeed again or ask for the bottle.

4. Some are fine at home but when at nursery or day care will be difficult and act out. Others are the opposite and are fine at nursery/day care but act out at home.

5. Some children are fine with the baby when they are young and immobile and once they start to move and grab or play with the siblings' toys intense feeling emerge.

As you can see every child is unique and will react to situations in different ways. It is important to know how to handle these situations.

Top Tips:

Try to avoid other major life events happening at the same time, for example moving house, starting nursery or toilet training.

Always try and reward your child for showing love and affection towards your baby whilst ignoring negative and babyish behaviour as far as possible (as long as it's not harmful to your baby. If your child shows any aggression towards your baby do not leave them alone together).

If your child does show open hostility to the baby tell them that the behaviour is wrong. Try not to make your child feel guilty about their actions. It is 'what' they are doing which is wrong and not them.

Chapter Eight – Sleep and Behaviour

Be careful about your language. Telling them they are 'good' or 'bad', labelling your child is not helpful and may harm them emotionally. Focus on the behaviour not the child.

Get your older child involved in your baby's care by asking them to get a nappy or cream for the baby. Don't push it if they don't want to as it will build up more resentment. But praise them if they are willing to help to encourage the desired behaviour.

Try and have some special one to one time with just you and your older child away from the baby.

Be observant towards your child. Watch for signs of being withdrawn or depressed, especially in older children. Intense feelings can be hard to deal with and they may need someone outside of the family to talk with.

Aggressive Behaviour

I think it is worth speaking more about aggressive behaviour as it is one of the harder behaviour issues that parents find the most challenging and upsetting. As with any behaviour problem the first step is prevention.

Prevention

It is important to lay out the ground rules before a baby arrives home so that your child is clear about what is and isn't expected of them. We do not want to set your child up for failure. These rules will be different in every household and you must be clear about them and consistent. For example, a simple rule may be that they never pick the baby up or only when the parent is in the room can the child hold or cuddle the baby. Another rule to protect the baby may be that they must never put anything in the baby's mouth (a dummy may be the exception to this rule). I have seen some children try and feed a new baby biscuits and ice cream, for example.

Help Them Learn Empathy

I have worked with children for many years and know that the key to discouraging aggressive behaviour is to help children learn to empathise with others. This can be taught from an early age. I have seen older sibling pinch and bite their new baby. This is so distressing for the parents and the new baby. But the parents' reaction is so crucial in how to manage this behaviour in order to stop it happening again. Empathy is the ability to understand how another person is feeling.

As parents, punishing your child for 'bad' behaviour will not prevent the 'bad' behaviour and it may even add to the problem. Instead teach the child how the baby feels. As, the baby can't talk the parent has to be their voice. Say to your child something like this 'do you remember when you fell over and cut your knee how it hurt? This gets your child in touch with their own feelings of hurt. Then say to them this is how your baby feels when you do X or Y. Point out to your child the baby's distress and that even though your baby can't speak they are telling you that 'it hurts' with their tears.

No matter how old your child is they will make the connection between their own hurt and the baby's hurt and this is how you build empathy in your child. In addition to helping them develop empathy, always give more attention to the hurt baby when dealing with aggressive behaviour in order to make your child's bid for attention fail. Make your child help with caring for the baby after by caring for the pinch or bite mark and this will show them the consequences of their actions. Use key words when caring for the baby like 'ouch' that

Chapter Eight – Sleep and Behaviour

looks very painful/sore and when comforting the baby say things like 'X is sorry for hurting you, he can see that you are hurting'. This is a very powerful way of a child learning to show empathy.

Always remember to reward your child for 'good' or desired behaviour. Undesired or 'bad' behaviour must *not* be ignored, especially aggressive behaviour. If the behaviour is more minor then another technique may be considered.

Redirection or Distraction

Many acts of 'bad behaviour' are simply attempts to get your attention. It is better to simply ignore *minor acts* of misbehaviour when dealing with toddler tantrums. If your child is acting out for attention then distraction or redirection is the best way forward. Simply get a toy or book out and draw the child's attention to this instead. Or look out the window and draw their attention elsewhere. Make it compelling for him and build his curiosity, he will be simply unable to resist. I particularly like the window distraction as it always worked for me. For example, say 'oh what's that boy doing' or 'quick X come and see there is an Y in the street' they will forget all about the tantrum and come running. Be careful not to use it too much and vary your distractions or they become desensitised to this technique. Always ensure that there is something exciting to draw them towards or they will get annoyed with you.

When dealing with unacceptable behaviour you need to take it up a step. As a psychologist I find behaviour and misbehaviour in children fascinating to work with. I love to teach parents about managing their children's behaviour as it is so easy to get it wrong and much harder to get it right.

Chapter Eight – Sleep and Behaviour

Positive Behaviour

Children will role model and copy their parents. We as parents are what we make our children, as we are their teachers. They will copy our words and our behaviours. We have a responsibility to teach them right and wrong. I always say to parents what are you teaching your child? Are you teaching them positive behaviour or negative behaviour? Do you reward 'good' behaviour or 'bad' behaviour?

If you want good behaviour you have to encourage good behaviour. So many times I see parents rewarding bad behaviour. I am in the supermarket and I see a child 'acting out' he wants to have some sweets and the mother gives in and buys the sweets. Let's look at what the child is learning from this parent. If I have a tantrum and cry I will get the sweets. Now I know it is difficult for parents if their child has a tantrum in the supermarket, they feel embarrassed and don't want to draw attention to themselves. So the mother rewards the bad behaviour with sweets. The child has learned that A = B. In this case if I cry and act out I will get the sweets. The mother reinforces this learning by giving him the sweets.

However, this behaviour may not have been rewarded if the child were at home. The child has learned that A=B and so he has a tantrum because he wants sweets. Now the mother when not being observed by shoppers takes a different action and decides not to give him the sweets. The child becomes confused as now he is doing the same behaviour but getting a different result - no sweets. But now A does not = B. The child is getting mixed messages and he persists in the hope he will get the result he wants and has learned previously. But now A equals something else. That something else may be a 'smack' or 'timeout' as the mother has lost her patience or is trying to deal with the unwanted behaviour.

Chapter Eight – Sleep and Behaviour

The above situation is very common in parenting. Every child needs consistency and continuity. They need rules and boundaries to feel safe and secure. You as parents must decide on the rules for your children and stick to them like glue to avoid confusing your child.

Tip # 12:

Reward desired behaviour and deal with the undesired behaviour. Be consistent and follow through on what you say.

Chapter Nine - Development

The Department of Health (DOH) has laid down their requirement of what developmental screening and surveillance should be carried out on children in England. This is delivered by HVs and is called the 'Healthy Child Programme' 2009.

Baby/Child Assessments/Developmental Checks

When health visitors carry out developmental assessments or checks we will use tools to help inform our judgements of where your baby/child is in their development. It guides professionals as to how to identify any deviation from normal healthy development. I will now give you an outline of what your baby should be achieving at each stage of their development.

Emotional/Intellectual Development

From birth your baby is totally dependent on you for food, warmth, comfort and love; we all know that of course. Your baby's brain has been physically growing since conception and will continue to grow throughout the nine months that you are pregnant. However, at birth the brain functions consist mainly of survival reflexes such as rooting and sucking for food, grasping, stepping, sleeping, crying – primary functions of the brain stem.

Your baby also has the ability to show emotions such as fear, affection, disgust and anger due to the early development of your baby's limbic

Chapter Nine - Development

system. Even at six weeks the cerebral cortex, the part of the brain responsible for thinking, feeling and memory, is still in the early stages of development. The knowledge that we now have about brain development has changed the old 'nature versus nurture' debate into a discussion about which genetic endowments will be expressed as a result of your baby's early childhood experiences. Is your baby born with natural abilities or are they affected by their environment? Psychologists like myself, find this a fascinating subject and we love to argue and debate this point. Babies do of course need good nutrition to grow and develop but equally important is love and stimulation from you the parents. Your baby is learning and growing from the day he or she is born, not only physically but emotionally too.

The newborn's brain is filled with sensory, motor, emotional and cognitive pathways ready to be shaped and modified based on every experience she has during the first few years of life. These experiences, from feeling your skin against theirs at birth to hearing the song you sing to them will when upset, will repeatedly stimulate and solidify some synapse or neural connections but not others. Those that are not used or stimulated will disappear.

This is a good thing as it means that the efficiency of the stimulated connections is increased and strengthened. For example, babies who grow up hearing their own language will develop connections to recognise only that language and will not be able to recognise others. So if you are a multilingual family I would suggest you speak in your native tongue as your baby will make these connections with ease. In this chapter I will focus on the development of language and hearing. Before babies speak they build up a huge store of knowledge about speech and language. This store of knowledge is called 'receptive speech'. When babies speak this is called 'expressive speech'.

Chapter Nine - Development

4 Weeks
At this young age your baby will have limited understanding. They will watch you closely when you are talking. Your baby will open and close their mouth as you speak and will go quite when they hear the sound of your voice.

6 Weeks
At six weeks your baby will follow your movements with their eyes and they will begin to smile at your voice. At six weeks your baby will startle, blink, cry and stop sucking when feeding on hearing sudden loud noises. The will also stop sucking or crying for a moment when you talk to them.

12 Weeks
At 12 weeks a baby will begin to grasp at objects of interest. They will smile frequently when spoken to and will begin to vocalise with gurgling noises to show pleasure.

16 Weeks
At 16 weeks your baby will have discovered their hands and will play with rattles for longer periods. At this age your baby will stir in their sleep to sudden loud noises. They will be soothed by your voice. Stop moving when there is a new sound. They will smile, coo, stop crying/sucking in response to your voice.

20 Weeks
At 20 weeks your baby will now be good at grasping objects. They will enjoy playing with toys. Bath time will be fun as they can now splash.

They are getting good at holding and discovering objects with their hands and activities like crumpling paper, they will enjoy the sound. They will start to recognise themselves in the mirror and smile at themselves. Sometimes if they drop a toy they will begin to look and see where it has gone.

24 Weeks

Your baby will now have discovered their feet and are now able to grasp them. Some may be able to hold their own bottle (not recommended). They will start to play games with you like peek-a-boo and around-the-garden. They will be smiling and vocalising at themselves in the mirror. If they drop a toy they will try and recover it for themselves. Your baby will imitate the faces you pull.

28 Weeks

By now your baby will be able to transfer an object/toy from one hand to another without it falling. They will reach out to pick up things with one hand instead of two. They will enjoy banging two objects together and everything will go into their mouth. They will still enjoy the sounds of crumpling paper. Your baby will now pat the face they see in the mirror. They will respond to their name when you call them. Your baby will imitate the faces you pull, for example, sticking out your tongue. If they don't get your attention they will cough or make noises to get what they want. They will be developing more sounds and the specific sound of 'da' 'ta' and 'ka'.

32 Weeks

From this age up until one year old your baby should be offered a developmental check by the health visiting service. This is primarily

Chapter Nine - Development

carried out around 8mts old and will be discussed in detail in the next paragraph. Development will be looked at under five headings;

Communication, Gross motor development, Fine motor development, Problem Solving and Personal-Social.

7-11 Month Developmental Check

This is an important milestone therefore I will be going into more detail as it is the next assessment to be carried out under 'The Healthy Child Programme'. It can be carried out at any stage from 8-12mts depending on your HV location and staff levels.

Physical Assessment

Your baby will have measurements taken. Height will range from 60cm (2 feet) 74cm (2.5 feet) with an average of 70cm (2 feet 3 inches). When weight and height is plotted on the percentile chart any measurement between these two readings will be considered within normal range. Weight will range from 6.5kg (14pounds 5 ounces) up to 11.5kg (25 pounds and 5 ounces) with an average of 8.5kg (18 pounds and 11 ounces).

Your baby will have their hips checked to ensure that they are stable. This is done by looking at the length of both legs. They should be equal in length and the skin creases matching on both sides. If leg length is unequal and the skin crease not matching this could indicate a problem with the hips and a referral would be suggested to the GP for further investigation.

In boys it is important to ensure that both testicles are down in the scrotum. In rare cases the testicles may not have descended or they could be 'retractile' which means that the testicle is normal but is pulled back out of the scrotum by a muscle reflex. If they have not been observed to be down at any stage then it is best to refer to the GP.

1. Communication

At 8 months old your baby should be doing the following;

When you are out of sight and call, your baby should look in the direction of your voice.

When your baby hears a loud noise they look to see where the sound came from.

When you copy the sounds your baby makes they should repeat the same sounds back to you.

Your baby should be making the following sounds "da," "ka," "ga" and "ba"

Your baby should respond to the tone of your voice and stop his activity at least briefly when you say "NO" to him.

Your baby should be able to make two similar sounds like "ba-ba," "da-da," or "ga-ga".

2. Gross Motor

Your baby should be sitting independently by now and should be able, when sitting on the floor, to lean forward on her hands for support.

Chapter Nine - Development

Most babies will be able to sit up straight for several minutes without using their hands for support.

Your baby should be rolling from his back and getting both arms out from under him.

Your baby should be able to stand upright on both feet whilst being supported by you holding onto his hands.

Your baby should be able to get into a crawling position by getting up on her hands and knees.

Your baby should be able to hold onto the bars of his cot and stand upright without needing to lean his chest against the cot for support.

3. Fine Motor

Your baby should be able reach out and pick up a 'cheerio' with her finger and thumb (pincer grasp).

Your baby should be able to pick up a small toy, holding it in the centre with his fingers around it.

Your baby should be able to pick up a toy using only one hand.

Your baby should be able to pick up a small toy with the tips of her thumb and fingers.

4. Problem Solving

Your baby should be able to pick up a toy and put it in his mouth.

When lying on her back, if she drops a toy she should try and get it if she can see it.

He should be able to bang a toy up and down on a surface.

Your baby should be able to pass a toy back and forward from one hand to another.

She should be able to pick up a toy in each hand and hold onto it for a second or two.

Your baby should be able to bang one toy against another toy.

5. Personal- Social

When your baby is lying on her back she should be able to grab her feet and play with them.

When in front of a mirror your baby should reach out and pat the mirror.

Your baby should be able to reach for a toy that is out of reach by rolling, pivoting or crawling.

Your baby should, when lying on his back, be able to put his foot in his mouth.

Your baby should be able to drink from a cup.

He should be able to feed himself a cracker or biscuit.

The next full developmental assessment will not be until your baby is 2 years old.

Chapter Nine - Development

36 Weeks
By now your baby will be using a pincher grasp picking up small objects with their finger and thumb rather than a palmer grasp- all fingers and thumb. Your baby should now turn his head towards sounds and enjoy musical toys and rattles. They will use their voice tunefully. They will take turns with you making sounds (having conversation) and will quieten when you speak from the next room or as you approach the room.

40 -42 Weeks
Your baby will now be able to reach out for toys and people. They will be able to pat a doll. They are beginning to understand single words in context and may be able to understand some body parts, name of self and family members. Your baby may pull on clothing to gain attention. They will start to wave bye-bye when you say the words or mimic the gesture. They will be saying one or two words with meaning.

48-52 Weeks
Your baby will now start to engage in play with you by giving and taking toys. They will enjoy repetitive games like putting bricks in a container and will show interest in books. They will delight in games like 'peek-a-boo'. Their understanding will be increasing and will understand the meaning of a range of common single words. They will also be saying one or more words with meaning.

13-15 Months
Your baby is now walking independently. He can make marks on paper with a pencil. And build a tower of two bricks. He will pat pictures of animals. He will gesture for things he wants by pointing. He will use lots of pretend talking.

18 Months

By now your toddler will be starting to run and climb. She can build a tower of three bricks, will use a spoon correctly and turn pages in a book two or three at time. She will enjoy scribbling and will copy common household tasks such as sweeping the floor or dusting. She will be able to point to a picture of everyday objects if asked and can point to her nose, eyes and head if asked. Will now be able to carry out two simple instructions like; get your coat and shoes. She will have an increasing vocabulary range of 0-6 single words and strings of 'pretend' speech. The sounds established will be p, b, m, n, and w. The sounds emerging are t, and d.

21 Months

Now your toddler will be better at manipulation and build a tower of five to six bricks. He will be able to point to body parts if asked and respond to his name. He will be able to pull people and points to show them objects. He will repeat things said to him. He will ask for food, drink and may know when he needs the toilet. He will have a vocabulary range of about 50 single words.

Chapter Nine - Development

2 Year Developmental Check

This will be the next formal assessment by the health visiting team under 'The Healthy Child Programme' and may be the last assessment carried out by the HV service if the development is progressing well and you the parent have no concerns.

Physical Check

Your toddler's height and weight measurements will again be taken. At 2 years your child height should be 80-96cm (2 feet 7.5inches- 3 feet i.8 inches) with an average of 88cm (2 feet 10.6inches). Weight should be 9-16kg (19 pounds and 13 ounces to 35 pounds and 3 ounces) with an average of 12kg (26 pounds and 6 ounces).

Gross Motor Development

Your child should by now be walking, running and climbing. They should be able to jump with both feet off the ground. They should have a dominant hand for drawing and eating. They should be able to kick a ball and be able to walk up or down two steps without holding on to a rail.

Fine Motor Development

They should be able to build a tower of six to seven bricks. They should be able to turn single pages of a book and able to put on shoes, socks and pants (although they may be in inside out or back to front). They should be able to copy straight lines and circles and hold a pencil with a pincher grasp.

Speech and Language

They should be able to put two together like 'all gone' and use words such as 'I', 'me', and 'you'. They should have a range of single words between; 50-100 (average range) and put 2 words together like 'me drink'. The sounds established will be; p, b, t, d, h, m, n, and w. The sounds emerging are; k, g, j, n, and g. They should be able to understand commands like 'find your coat' or 'take my hand'. They will repeat words you say.

Problem Solving

Your child should be able to line up four blocks or cars in a row. If something is out of their reach on a ledge or surface they will now get a chair and climb on it to get what they want. They should know where things belong and be able to put them back in their rightful place. They should be using pretend play and using their imagination, for example, holding an object to their ear and pretending to speak on the telephone.

Personal Social

Your child should be able to drink out of a cup without spilling it and eat with a fork. They should be using pretend play like feeding or changing the doll. They should be able to push a pram or other toy with wheels, steering it around objects.

This is a good age to start thinking about putting your child down for a nursery place. Some children will be entitled to a free nursery place up to 15hrs per week if the family is in receipt of any benefits (this will depend on the area that you live).

Personality

By now your child will have developed their own unique personality. At 2yrs old they are very ego centric, so everything will centre on and around them. They will be very strong willed and will often say words like 'me do it' or 'I do it'. If your child does not get want they want they will 'act out'. This is the time of the temper tantrums and you will need all your resources to manage behaviour issues.

Children of all ages will need firm boundaries and you as parents will need to have a plan of how to manage behaviour issues. The first thing you need to agree on is what is acceptable and unacceptable for you as parents. Sometimes something may be acceptable to one parent and not the other. This is a tricky situation as children need consistency and continuity. You will *both* have to decide on how to manage behaviour that is not acceptable. For example, if one parent doesn't like a child being up until 10pm and watching kids T.V and the other simply does not see this as an issue then you have a problem. So you may want to talk about your 'family rules', what will and will not happen in your house. Once you have agreed then you STICK with the rules. It is so important that you both follow through on your rules. If bed time is 7pm then it should be 7pm each and every evening. Children need to know that both mum and dad are singing from the same hymn book, if not it will lead to confusion and lots of tension in the household.

(See more on parenting style in Chapter 11)

Toilet Training

Between 2 and 2.5 years your child should be showing some signs of being ready for toilet training. One of the first signs is to know or have some understanding when they are wet or dirty. Some children may well be dry by 2years but many will not be.

Personal story

When I was toilet training my first son I started him when I wanted him to train at 2yrs rather than waiting until he was ready. I made this decision as I had two children in nappies and besides being hard work (as I seemed to be changing nappies all day), it was also expensive. It was a nightmare. He had no idea what to do. He would sit on the potty but do nothing and as soon as he came off he would wee on the floor and think it was funny. We went through hundreds of wet pants each week and that went on for a year. It was complicated by him having an operation half way through the training. He didn't get dry until a week before his third birthday. I certainly learned from that negative experience as I spent a year being stressed out.

I don't recommend toilet training until your child is showing signs of readiness:

Bladder control; having a gap between wetting of at least an hour up (to 2hrs is preferable).

They know when they are passing urine and may tell you.

Emotional readiness; being able to obey commands and have understanding.

Chapter Nine - Development

Avoid starting when there is a new baby in the house or any other major life change.

Physical readiness- being able to pull pants/pull ups up and down.

Every child is different and my second child trained in a couple of weeks having left him until two and half years to train. It is best not to compare your child with someone else's. Most children by the age of two years are dry by day and most will be dry by night six to 12 months later. The majority of children will gain bowel control first before gaining bladder control and this is more predictable and regular in pattern. By the age of three years, 9 out of 10 children will be dry by day but may be still wetting at night and have the occasional accident. By the age of four most children are reliably dry. If your child is not dry by this age go and see your GP or HV to make sure there is no underlying medical reason.

Sometimes, in a previously dry child, they can regress back if they are under any stress as mentioned earlier (the arrival of a baby, starting nursery, moving house). This is to be expected and is normal; it will soon sort itself out.

2 ½ Years

By now your child can build a tower of eight bricks and will copy drawing lines on paper. They will begin to seek adult involvement in their play, for example, making cups of tea, putting the baby to bed. They will enjoy imitating others play. Your child will be able to, understand instructions with 2-3 key words in and will also understand the function of some objects, for example, the washing machine is for washing clothes. Most will be able to match colours and some will recognise the primary colours. They should be able to count to 10 but some will go beyond and may reach 20 but not in sequence.

They will be able to ask questions to initiate conversations. You will constantly hear the words 'What's that?'. They should have a vocabulary of between 50-200 words and will know object names, names of people, action names, along with 'what', 'where', 'here'. They will be stringing words together like 'goodbye daddy'. They will also use 2-3 word phrases like; 'daddy gone work'. The sounds established will be; p, b, t, d, k, g, h, m, n, w, and j. The sounds emerging will be f, s, and l.

3 Years

By this age your child will be able to build a tower of nine bricks and be able to dress and undress themselves but will still need help with buttons and fasteners. They will now be getting the shoes on the right feet and know the back and front of clothes. They will be able to copy a circle and cross on paper and may even be spontaneously drawing a face with eyes, nose and mouth with arms and legs coming from the face.

They will join in with others during play and be more interactive. They will now know their own sex. They will know the difference between 'on' 'in', and 'under' and will understand basic concepts like big and little, happy and sad. They will sing nursery rhymes. They should be able to count to 10, some will go beyond this. They will know primary and some secondary colours. They will have a vocabulary of 200+ words and be using 3 word phrases including questions beginning with 'who' 'what'. They will be constantly continuing to ask questions. They may be able to use the past tense 'I went' or 'I done it'. They will be able to comment on events and take part in short conversations. Sometimes they will have difficulty with the beginning of blend letters like chair or shout and will drop off the blend and instead say 'air' or 'out', this is quite normal. As well as having difficulty with double consonants they may sometimes use letter substitutions. Instead of saying 'car' they may say 'tar' again this is normal at this age. This may not disappear until they are older.

3-4 years

By now your child's gross motor development will be increasing. They will be able to pedal a tricycle. Their concentration will be also increasing and they will now be able to sustain play on their own. They will use their imagination more and start using symbolic play pretending they are spacemen and driving a rocket into space and will talk to themselves in play. They will enjoy interacting with their peers for short periods. They will now be using 3-4 key word instructions and understand more complex grammatical sentence structures. They will have a large vocabulary including names, actions, place words and basic concept words (colour, shape and size). They will use 4+ word phrases like 'I go home now '. They will continue to ask questions, but they will now introduce the 'how' and 'why' of things. They will start to use plurals but will add 'S' to the singular like 'mouse's instead of 'mice' or put 'ed' for everything in the past tense for example 'breaked' instead of 'broke' .

They will take turns in conversation and will try and make themselves understood if the listener has not quite understood them. The sounds established are p, b, t, d, k, g, h, v, f, s, z, sh, m, n, w, l, and j. The sounds emerging are ch, s-clusters, l-blends and r-blends.

4-5 Years

By now you should be encouraging your child to be independent in dressing and undressing in preparation for school. They should be able to do up buttons and zips and learning to tie shoe laces. They should be able to jump, skip and hop. They will be able to participate in group activities, listen to others and take turns. They should be able to understand simple rules to games and stick to them. They will enjoy operative play like the home corner/dressing up. Their understanding will be increasing and now they will now understand 4+ key word instructions and a variety of complex sentences. They will now be able to understand category names for words, for example, fruit.

Their vocabulary will be wide and include abstract concepts and things outside their experience. They will continue to ask questions and will be able to link ideas using long and complex sentences. They will be able to reason with you and will try and get out of things like going to bed for example. They will now be introducing words like but, because, so, and if into their sentences. They will also start to understand humour and use jokes. They will now have all the sounds in the alphabet except 'r' 'th' and 'J' which will emerge later.

Bonus Chapter One

Chapter Ten - The Theory and Practice of Learning and Development

Neuroscience

Your baby learns by forming connections in the brain. These are like building blocks, repetition will help this process. There are several theories to learning and this approach is what psychologist's name *'scaffolding'*. It is of course important to play with your baby and give them as many opportunities to learn as possible. The psychologist who termed this phrase is named Vygotsky. He believed, as I do, that in this type of learning the adult controls some elements of the situation sufficiently to allow the infant to make progress and to achieve results in a way that they would be unable to do alone. The Early Stage Foundation Stage (EYFS) Curriculum is based around this theory and is what is implemented in nurseries and schools.

Psychological Development

There are many theories surrounding psychological development which I have studied as a psychologist. But this is not a book on psychology so I will just give a small introduction into the four main approaches.

Chapter Ten: The Theory and Practice of Learning and Development

Behaviourism

A very famous psychologist named 'Skinner' came up with the behaviourist approach. His theory is based on the premise that babies and children learn from previous behaviours. If you reward the good behaviour it will continue. If you reward the undesired behaviour, then that behaviour will continue. But if you punish the 'bad' behaviour then the 'bad' behaviour will cease.

To illustrate this point, when I teach sleep training I sometimes use this in my teaching approach. For example, if a child learns to go to sleep, whether it be on the breast, holding mothers hand or lying beside their mother. This is learned behaviour and when repeated on a regular basis, this behaviour is reinforced through the parents. The child becomes conditioned to this behaviour. This means that the child is unable to go to sleep by themselves. He is conditioned to a certain way a 'learned behaviour'. When the parent wants to break the negative or undesired behaviour, the child understandably rebels by crying/acting out.

In order to get rid of the 'bad' or undesired behaviour the child has to unlearn the behaviour and learn another strategy a discussed in my chapter on sleep.

Social Learning Theory

This approach is based around the concept of children learning by watching the people around them. The sad fact is that our children will be a product of what they have observed and been taught by us. A Psychologist named 'Albert Bandura' carried out some experiments with children. Some children watched a video of a man being aggressive towards a 'dummy' person and his behaviour was rewarded.

Chapter Ten: The Theory and Practice of Learning and Development

Another group watched the same video but on this occasion the man was punished for his actions.

A third group of children who watched the film did not see any consequences for the behaviour. Following the film, the children were observed in how they would react towards a 'dummy' doll when left alone in the room. Those who had seen the man punished for his actions were much less likely to act with aggression towards the doll than the other two groups.

So we can see that children do learn, from the outcomes of how their behaviour is managed. This is learned at a young age during the child's imprinting period. How they behave as children will be how they behave as adults.

Constructivism

Jean Piaget came up with his four stage theory of development.

Stage 1: Sensory – motor (from birth to about 2years)

Children learn through their senses, to make sense of their world. Small babies will put everything in their mouth this is how they learn.

Stage 2: Pre-operational stage (from about 2 to 6 years)

This is when children begin to put connections together to make sense of the world. For example, putting two objects together can be represented symbolically as an abstract mathematical principle (addition).

Stage 3: Concrete operations stage (from about 6 to 12 years)

At this stage of development children are interacting and socialising with the world around them. They develop the ability to generate 'rules' based on their own experiences. They are still only able to understand the rules that they have had concrete experience of, but can now begin some mental manipulation of these concepts. What they are unable to do at this stage is use rules to anticipate something that could happen, but that they have not yet experienced.

Stage 4: Formal operations (from about 12years onwards)

By this stage children can reason in a purely abstract way, without reference to concrete experience.

Social Constructivism

'Vygotskys' approach was simpler he felt that human history and development was created through 'cultural tools' the most important of these being language.

Although psychologists will argue from their own perspective what they all agree on, is how rapid the child will grow and learn from birth. This first year of development is crucial as this is when your baby's brain is growing at a rapid rate. Your baby's cerebral cortex will triple in thickness in her first year of life and by the time she is 18months old her brain will weigh almost two-thirds of its eventual adult weight. The hundred billion neurons a baby is born with, over the next several years will undergo an amazing process of synaptic connection to build and strengthen the neurons into a complex network of nerve pathways just like a super highway.

The brain is an experience dependent organ, and during this massive period of growth your baby's brain is more receptive to learning through nurturing, enriching experiences than at any other time of her development. The more you stimulate and play with your baby the better chance she has of reaching normal developmental milestones. Conversely, it is also a time of great vulnerability, when a lack of nurturing and lack of stimulation can compromise her potential.

Neuroscience is extremely relevant information in helping us to understand learning and early development. With new technologies that allow us to see what learning looks like, we have new information about the way the brain develops and the neurological and biological 'pathways' that affect the way we develop throughout life.

We now have a new understanding of how sensory stimulation, such as touch, vision, sound, taste, smell, pain, temperature and positioning affect the structure of and function of the brain during early development. When a baby receives stimuli through the sense organs billions of connections are being made, these connections are called synapses. This is most active in utero and the following 3 yrs of development.

These early years are the most precious and can make a tremendous difference to the child's cognitive ability. There has been a shift in the way psychologists have viewed learning and development.

Past Thinking:

How the brain develops depends on the genes you were born with.

The experiences you have before age three have a limited impact in later development.

The secure relationship with a primary care giver creates a favourable context for early development and learning.

Chapter Ten: The Theory and Practice of Learning and Development

Brain development is linear. The brain's capacity to learn and change grows steadily as the infant progresses toward adulthood.

A toddler's brain is much less active than of a university student.

Present Thinking

How a brain develops depends on a complex interplay between the genes you are born with and the experiences you have.

Early experiences have a decisive impact on the architecture of the brain and on nature and the extent of the adult capacities.

Early interactions don't just create a context; they directly affect the way the brain is 'wired'.

Brain development is not-linear; there are prime times for acquiring different kinds of knowledge and skills. You may notice that your baby goes through 'sensitive' periods where they become almost obsessed by a certain toy or activity and they will keep repeating this activity as it gives them great satisfaction.

By the time children reach age three, their brains are twice as active as those of adults. Activity level drops during adolescence.

The next section will cover some suggested ways to help stimulate your baby's development and hence maximise your child's potential in life.

Chapter Ten: The Theory and Practice of Learning and Development

How Can You Stimulate Your Baby in the Five Areas of Development?

Activities for Babies 8-12 Months Old

Communication

Read baby books or colourful magazines by pointing and telling your baby what is in the picture. Let your baby pat pictures in the book.

Point to pictures in the book and say the word. Repeat this word so your baby can learn to associate the picture with that word.

Read the same book at regular intervals to reinforce the learning.

Speak to your baby at every opportunity; allow pauses in between, this will allow your baby to respond. This is a vital learning for your baby and teaches them about how conversations work.

Say 'hello' and wave when entering a room with your baby and make the gesture of raising your hand. Help your baby to raise their hand and wave 'bye' when leaving a room.

Attend 'story time' or 'singing time' at your local library. Babies will love the action songs and this will build up their understanding of language.

Fine Motor

Your baby will enjoy banging objects together that make a noise; they do not have to be expensive shop bought toys. Baby's love everyday household items to play with. I always found pots and pans to be the most fun and exciting. Join in and show your baby how to have fun.

Give your baby blocks to bang, rattles to shake, or wooden spoons to bang on the pots and pans.

A good pastime is putting objects in and out of containers. Give your baby opportunities to do this by getting them to post dry pasta shapes into plastic bottles with small openings.

Get your baby to pass objects from one shoebox into another again just make the hole big enough to accommodate the objects chosen. Choose larger objects for younger baby's and gradually make the objects smaller, like beads or dry beans (always observe your baby as they play with smaller objects).

As your baby gets older he will begin to use his index finger to poke or pick things up with a pincer grip-finger and thumb. Use objects like telephones with buttons that invite poking. Your baby may poke you in the face. Use this opportunity to name body parts on your face. Play games like head, shoulders, knees and toes'.

Gross Motor

Put toys beside or in front of your baby to encourage them to roll over and crawl forward. Use your voice to encourage them to move.

Put toys on the sofa or sturdy table so that your baby can practice standing while playing with toys.

Find a big box that your baby can crawl in and out of. Stay close by and talk to your baby about what she is doing. "You went in!" "Now you are out!"

Chapter Ten: The Theory and Practice of Learning and Development

Play ball games. Roll a ball to your baby. Help your baby, or have a partner help him roll the ball back to you. Your baby may even throw the ball, so make sure they are nice and soft.

Let your baby play with soft plastic measuring cups, cups with handles, sieves, strainers, sponges, and balls that float in the bath. Bath time is a great time for learning.

Problem Solving

Play hide-and-seek games with objects. Let your baby see you hide an object under a cloth, nappy, or pillow. If your baby doesn't uncover the object, just cover part of it. Help your baby find the object.

Play 'pat-a-cake' with your baby clap hands together or take turns. Wait and see if your baby signals you to start the game again. Try the game using blocks or spoons to clap and bang with.

Make a simple puzzle for your baby by putting blocks or ping pong balls inside a muffin tray or egg carton. See if your baby can lift them out.

You can make a simple toy by cutting a hole in the plastic lid of a coffee jar. Give your baby wooden clothes pegs or ping pong balls to drop inside.

Let your baby makes choices. Offer two toys or foods and see which one your baby picks. Encourage your baby to reach or point to the chosen object. Babies have definite likes and dislikes.

Chapter Ten: The Theory and Practice of Learning and Development

Personal Social

Mirrors are exciting at this age. Let your baby pat and poke at herself in the mirror. Smile and make faces together in the mirror.

Play imitation games like peek-a-boo and round-the –garden. Show pleasure at your baby's imitations of movements and sounds. Babies enjoy playing the same games over and over.

Make sure you take your baby to mother and toddler groups and use every opportunity to socialise with your baby.

Talk to your baby at every opportunity, allowing them to 'make conversation' with you. Give them time to answer by the use of frequent pausing.

Most of all have fun with your baby, sing, read, dance and be silly in your behaviour with your baby.

Activities for Children 24-30 Months old

Communication

Speak and read to your with your child at every opportunity.

Add an old magazine/catalogue or two to your child's library. It's a good 'picture' book for naming common objects.

Add actions to your child's favourite nursery rhymes. Easy action rhymes include 'The wheels on the bus' Row, Row, Row, your boat' and 'if your happy and you know it'.

Action is important part of a child's life. Play a game with a ball where you give directions and your child does the actions, such as 'roll the

Chapter Ten: The Theory and Practice of Learning and Development

ball', kick; throw, bounce and catch are other good action words. Take turns giving the directions.

Make an obstacle course using chairs, pillows, or large boxes. Tell your child to crawl over, under, through, behind, in front of, or between the objects. Be careful arranging the pieces so that your child doesn't fall and hurt themselves.

Fine Motor

Get your toddler to spoon rice from one bowl into another or pour water from one plastic jug to another. These types of activities will encourage hand eye co-ordination.

Get an assortment of jars and get your toddler to open and close the lids.

Get various sizes of locks and keys and see if your toddler can and open the lock.

Take time to draw with your child when she wants to get out paper and crayons. Draw large shapes and let your child colour them in. Take turns.

Try a new twist to finger painting. Use whipping cream or shaving foam on a washable surface. Help your child to spread it around and draw pictures with your fingers. Add food colouring if you want to give it some colour.

Gross Motor

Play 'follow the leader 'walk on tiptoes, walk backwards, and walk slow or fast with big steps and little steps.

Chapter Ten: The Theory and Practice of Learning and Development

Play target toss with a large bucket or box and bean bags or balls. Help your child count how many she gets in the target. A ball of wool or rolled up socks also work well for indoor target practice.

Play a jumping game when you take a walk by jumping over the cracks in the pavement. You may have to hold your child's hand and help him jump at first.

Enhance listening skills by playing music with both slow and fast rhythms. Songs with speed changes are great. Show your child how to move fast or slow with the music.

Make an obstacle course using chairs, pillows, or large boxes. Tell your child to crawl over, under, through, behind, in front of, or between the objects. Be careful arranging the pieces so that your child doesn't fall and hurt themselves.

Problem Solving

Collect little and big things around the house. Show and describe (big/little) the objects. Ask your child to give you the big ball, then all of the big balls. Do the same for little.

Another big/little game is making yourself big by stretching your arms up high and making yourself little by squatting. Ask your child, if there is other ways they can make themselves big/small.

Make sound containers using empty plastic bottles. Use different substances, like rice, beans, or coins, and part fill them. Make two of each type. When you shake them ask your child which ones make the same noise and which ones are different. You can take this a step further asking your child questions like 'does this make a higher/lower sound' or 'is this one heavier/lighter' etc.

Chapter Ten: The Theory and Practice of Learning and Development

Tasting/smelling games can be fun. If your child is happy to be blindfolded you can guess the smell or taste of different household foods like fruits or vegetables (this can be particularly good if a child dislikes a taste sometimes it can be revealing to them that in fact they do like that particular taste).

Place a number of items on a tray and then, let your child to spend time carefully looking at the tray. Remove one item from the tray and ask your child, if they can they can spot the missing item. Use only a small amount of items at first and then build it up as your child build confidence.

Personal Social

Give your child soap, a washcloth, and a bowl of water. Let your child wash a 'dirty' doll, toy dishes, or doll clothes. It's good practice for hand washing and drying.

Get your child to fold clothes with you from the dryer, or pair socks together.

Get your child to help with setting the table. Putting the knives, and forks, cups and, place mats, on the table. Get them to count out the number of each item as you do it together.

Let your child help get themselves dressed/undressed in the morning and evenings. They should be able to manage socks, shoes, coat, and hat.

Children love going on outings. One special outing can be the library to meet other children for story/singing time. You could also go to mother and toddler groups. Mixing with other children and joining in will help with developing social skills like turn taking.

Chapter Ten: The Theory and Practice of Learning and Development

Summary

Psychological child development is so important in children. I cover the theories only to give you more information and knowledge in this area.

If you look at development overall we can view it in the following ways:

Development as a discipline – behaviourism.

Development as an experience – social learning theory.

Development as 'natural stages' – constructivism.

Development as interaction – social constructivism.

In reality when I work with families I will bring in all this knowledge. I feel the theories cannot be looked at in isolation as they all impact on one another when it comes to child's emotional and psychological well-being and development.

Bonus Chapter Two

Chapter Eleven - The Importance of Parenting

Why did you Become a Parent?

Have you ever stopped to think of why you wanted to become a parent or what kind of a parent you would most like to be? What are your strengths, your challenges? How has your childhood, religion, school, friends, culture and experience of being parented shaped you? These are all important questions to ask yourself before you become a parent but few of us, including myself ever do.

What is a Parent?

In its most limited, biological sense, being a parent is simply the business of contributing a set of chromosomes to a fertilized egg, thus becoming a 'biological parent'. In modern day life many women are bringing up children on their own without the fathers, some out of choice and others not from choice. But we all know there is much more to being a parent than the physical act of intercourse. To be a parent is a lifelong commitment for better or worse, as they say in the marriage vows. However, children can't divorce their parents (unless you are American of course then anything is possible) and parents can't divorce their children. However, we know from the media that many simply opt out of parenting when the going gets tough or, in some extreme cases, the parent may be in want of a night out or a holiday and leave their children home alone to fend for themselves.

As women, we cannot walk away after intercourse. We have to deal with the consequences and the reality that this may bring to our lives.

Chapter Eleven – The Importance of Parenting

Many know the risks but still take the chance of becoming pregnant. If we decide to commit to being a mother then there are a further nine months of pregnancy, supporting the growth of the baby not to mention the pain of labour and birth. In the majority of cases it will be the mother who will be the primary caregiver and nurturer of the baby and hopefully supported of her partner/husband and other family members.

Why is Parenting Important?

In modern culture parenting is widely thought of as an essential contribution to the development of personality- that is to say all the characteristics that make you and me who we are. It will determine how we relate with our partners and family members. There is much responsibility on us as parents. The specific qualities of relationships between parents and their children are commonly held to account for both positive and negative outcomes for children in the development of their personality. In other words we shape our children's personalities, I have mentioned this before but it is so important and worth mentioning again.

Successful people often praise the support and guidance of their parents in their formative years. Sadly, the opposite is true in cases of criminal behaviour. Many 'blame' their actions on their parents. I have certainly seen the effects of 'good' and 'poor' parenting in my 20 yrs as a health visitor. However, the good news is that we don't have to be perfect; *'good enough'* is just fine.

Chapter Eleven – The Importance of Parenting

The Importance of Parenting in the Early Years

So we know that early parenting is important. Strong attachment between a mother and her baby is crucial for physical and emotional development. The first three years of a child's life will affect all the rest.

When I was training as a Montessori Teacher one of the many books I read by Maria Montessori was called the 'Secret of Childhood'. In it she states the following statement which I find very profound even to this day:

"Show me the child at 3years old and I will show you the man".

She believed way back in 1949, that the impact of the first few years on a child's life had a lasting effect on the child's subsequent personality and behaviour. Her view of course is echoed by numerous psychologists around the world both before her and after her. From most psychological perspectives, parents are seen as the primary agents who constrain, organise and structure their children's experiences and personalities.

A dominant concern is that poor parenting results in children lacking the key skills that they need to adequately raise their own children to be able to function as well, adjusted members of society.

What Type of Parent Are You?

There are basically three types of parents:

1. Authoritarian

Authoritarian parenting has also been called military style parenting or aggressive parenting. This is because this style of parenting is

Chapter Eleven – The Importance of Parenting

demanding and not as much about a healthy development of the child as it is about rules, boundaries, and distance. In this form of parenting, parents do not encourage talking about feelings or stepping outside the boundaries. Children are expected to be completely dominated by their parents; much like the military is with its active service men and women.

The main goal of authoritarian parenting is to provide children with a strict set of rules that generally change as the child gets older and then the parenting becomes much stricter. Physical punishments are common in this approach, with some children suffering from abuse. The idea is to have control and shape children through instilling respect through fear and not stepping out of line. There is little room for arguments or flexibility; what is said the first time goes for every single time.

2. Permissive Parenting

Permissive parenting is the opposite of the authoritarian approach. Permissive parents want their children to be as free as possible; they want to be a friend to their children rather than a parent. There are no expectations or defined boundaries for the behaviour of their children. Children please themselves when they eat, what they eat, what time they go to bed, when they come home. The parents opt to warmly and lovingly accept however their offspring behave. They believe that giving and showing a child love, and getting loved back, is what parenting is all about.

Children of permissive parents are given as many options as possible, no matter how bad their decision-making abilities are. Discipline does not exist within a permissive household. Parents who employ permissive parenting get their children to act or follow loose rules with the use of gifts, bribes or any other means of conflict-less motivation.

3. Democratic Parenting

Democratic parenting involves a lot of communication and mutual understanding from both you the parent and your child. There will be rules and regulations which your child has to follow, but you do listen and let them speak their minds. When you tell them wrong, you as parents will be sure to give them the reason of why it is wrong and unacceptable.

If there is going to be punishment involved, you as parents will make sure your child knows why. This type of parenting brings everyone together. This type of parenting gives children respect and they will reciprocate. Together with your child you will be able to handle conflicts in a better way. If your child is right and you are wrong – you will be big enough to admit you were wrong and say sorry. It is alright for parents to be wrong sometimes, it shows that you are human too and sometimes make mistakes.

Your children will learn to think by themselves while being monitored by you their parents. You are not limiting their creativity, mind, thoughts and passions in any way. You are simply guiding them. They will learn to become dependent within the boundaries that you have set for them. This makes for happy healthy relationships.

Positive Parenting

What is positive parenting?

Chapter Eleven – The Importance of Parenting

Positive parenting is raising your children to be good citizens of the future, to have good moral judgement, values and ethics; to treat others with the respect. The best gift that you can give your children is love and respect. If your child is shown love and respect as children they will be able to give to others in adulthood. By giving your child the resources to grow knowing they are loved will give them a sense of value. If they are loved and valued they will grow up with high self-esteem, confidence and security to go out in the world and achieve their best. You as the parent have an enormous duty to shape your children into who they will become as adults. The interactions you choose to have with your child will be shaped from the moment they are born and will have a huge impact on the relationship you will have with them. So it is worth paying some attention to how the attachment of the mother to her child can influence the behaviour of the child.

Attachment Theory

In the first year of life, infants depend on their primary carers for food, warmth and affection, and therefore must be able to trust completely that their primary carers will provide these for them. If their needs are consistently met and responded to then they will develop a strong and secure attachment which is then repeated in their own parenting.

However, those infants whose needs are not consistently met, ignored all together or only met after unbearable pain by delaying them their basic needs will develop insecure attachments. A psychologist named Ainsworth developed an experiment on attachment called – 'Strange Situation'. She found that infants behaved in two distinct ways secure and insecure. The insecure attachments were further subdivided into; insecure resistant/ambivalent and insecure avoidant.

Secure Attachment

In her studies Ainsworth was looking at three things, how babies reacted when;

1. A stranger entered the room.

2. When their mother left the room.

3. When the mother returned to the room.

In a healthy attachment, babies should use the mother as a secure base, so when a stranger enters the room the baby should move nearer the parent for security. When the mother leaves the room, the baby should show natural concern, by crying or searching for her. When the mother returns to the room the baby will be eager to greet her and look for comfort. This group were known as the secure group or Type B.

Insecure Attachment

However, some babies did not use their mother as a secure base they seemed unwilling to seek comfort, these were called insecure. When their mothers left the room they were distressed but when the mother re-entered the room the babies' seemed to be ambivalent towards her, hence the term, insecure-ambivalent or Type C.

The remainder of babies in this insecure group showed concern when the mother left the room, however, on her return they actively avoided or ignored the parent. This group is known as the insecure avoidant – Type A.

A fourth group, Type D, was added to this in 1990. These infants showed contradictory behaviour patterns, at the same time and incomplete or undirected movements, and they seemed to be confused or apprehensive about approaching their parents. They appeared to be disorganised or disorientated in their behaviour.

The Importance of Knowing Your Baby's Personality

When you play with your baby/child you are literally helping to grow and expand their brain by interacting with them. Neurotransmitters are being released at the synaptic junctions. When your baby touches something or tastes something for the first time more connections are being made. According to Maria Montessori every baby will go through *'sensitive periods'* when they are almost obsessed with a certain toy or sound. A mother needs to notice these times. If you see your baby taking a special interest in something, allow him to look at it closely for as long as he wishes. Lift him up to the level at which his gaze is fixed and see his face light up with interest and love for whatever it was that drew his attention. When considering play activities for your baby/child it is important to first consider their personality or temperament. Not all activities are right for your child. You need to find the right one for them. So let us look at different personality types.

Chapter Eleven – The Importance of Parenting

Temperament

Your baby/child is unique and each baby will need to be treated in a different way. Are some babies/children just easier to get along with and to a parent? Temperament is one's character or disposition and all babies are different with their own unique personality. There are basically nine different traits observed in babies. Babies can react in a positive of negative manner in their traits.

1. First Reactions (FR)–Approach or Withdrawal. This is how a baby will react when first coming into contact with a new person, place or thing. A baby who is positive in FR will smile, reach out and not be afraid to welcome newness. A baby who is negative will be cautious maybe cry or cuddle up to their mother for protection.

Baby

These babies prefer to be in a safer or more familiar environment, like the home. This may lead to a mother staying at home in order to meet the needs of her baby/child's personality. Baby's positive in first reactions will be happy to go out and attend mother and toddler groups or meet with your friends for coffee or lunch. They are good with family members and don't mind being left with different people. On the other hand, babies who are negative in first reactions are a bit more cautious and shy when it comes to mixing with lots of people.

Child

Positive:

- These children are attracted to new things whether safe or dangerous.
- Readily makes and visits new friends

Negative:

- Hates new nurseries/groups/schools
- Hates new teacher
- Does not want to go to a new friend's house
- Is cautious in making new friends

2. Adaptability -this is the ease with which a baby will adapt to change. A baby who is high in adaptability will not mind his routine being changed and will sleep or eat at any time. A baby low in adaptability will find change difficult to cope with and fuss in a new environment.

Babies that are high in adaptability are quite social and don't mind if they miss out on a nap time or feeding time. They will simply grab a nap on the way to wherever you are going and pretty much fit in with your routine. Lucky you!

However, those babies who are lower in adaptability will struggle with challenges in routine. They like to be fed at regular intervals and need to have regular naps. They will not take kindly to being disrupted in their routines.

Child

High:

- Goes with the flow
- Easily adjusts to new bed when on holiday
- Moves easily from playing to sitting down for dinner

Low:

- Takes time settling in

- Gets very upset when family plans change
- Difficulty with disappointment

3. Mood - this is about how a baby approaches life in a positive way or a negative way (glass half full/empty). A baby with a high mood will be of a sunny disposition and smile a lot. A baby who is low in mood will be the opposite and be more demanding.

If your baby is high in mood they are normally happy to be around you, your family and friends. They are quite 'chilled out' and rarely cry, unless they have good reason to of course. Some people might label these baby's as a 'good' baby because they are not demanding of your time they will often amuse themselves. However, if your baby is low in mood they may be more challenging and need more attention as they will cry more and want to be held. Sadly, these babies are often labelled as 'naughty' babies. Some mothers will avoid going out as they fear their child will not 'behave' in public. Of course this is reinforced by the public in giving the mother accusing looks. This often causes the mother to stay at home where she feels safe and not judged.

Child

Positive:

- Smiles a lot
- Is outgoing and optimistic

Negative:

- Has more serious expression when meeting new people
- May whine or complain a lot
- Often appears to be dreaming or in a serious thought

Chapter Eleven – The Importance of Parenting

4. Activity level - this is how much a baby will move around. If high in activity level a baby will be constantly on the move and never sit still. If low in activity level then they are happy just to sit and relax.

Babies high in activity love to be on the go, they rarely sleep and can be a challenge to a sleep deprived mother. They will catch forty winks and then they are ready for action. They will demand your time and be into everything, you will need eyes in the back of your head as these are the babies that end up getting into difficulty. Danger sometimes follows them around and they will be the ones ending up with cuts and bruises and more. The minute you take your eyes off them they will find themselves in trouble. These babies love to play rough and tumble with their older siblings or father. Babies who are low in activity level are quite happy just to sit quietly on your lap or in a chair. They are content with quieter activities like reading or singing.

Child

High:

- Afterschool/nursery will want to go out and play an active game or sport

Low:

- Will quietly work on a puzzle or read a book

5. Intensity this is the degree of energy a baby has. If high then he may cry and or laugh a lot. If low, quite or mellow they may fuss rather than cry and smile rather than laugh.

Babies that are high in intensity don't do anything by halves. When they are happy everyone will know it, as they will heard, laughing out loud. If they are sad or angry they will also let you know it as they will be scream at you to make their feelings known. These babies will go from happy to sad in a short period of time and you may be in for a bit of roller coaster ride. Try and read the cues to prevent their emotions reaching its peak anticipate their needs. For example, if it's getting near to feeding time make sure you have food at hand, after all you don't want to scare the neighbours'. If your baby is lower in intensity they will be prepared to wait a little longer for their food or nap. They are a little more flexible with their needs.

Child

High:

- Situations are either great or horrible
- Has no middle ground
- Is more difficult to live with

Low:

- Is more predictable in reactions
- Is more subtle in responses
- May be incorrectly seen as being unenthusiastic
- Is easier to live with

6. Sensitivity is the level of sensory stimulation required to get a reaction. Some babies with high sensitivity are more aware of their surroundings; react quickly to changes in noise, temperature, texture and handling. Those with low sensitivity are less likely to react to noises and will not mind being in wet or dirty nappy.

Babies who are high in sensitivity need careful handling if they are to feel safe. They like people to speak softly to them and don't like any kind of rough activities. They like to be surrounded in peace and harmony from the clothes you put on them to the way you handle them. They are like a piece of expensive china and are easily broken, both verbally and physically. The baby who is low in sensitivity is the opposite, they don't mind if you shout or raise your voice or handle them roughly. They are more robust and can handle noisier or busier households.

Child

High:

- Complains of socks being too tight, or the label on the back of shirts scratching
- Notices emotions on people's faces
- May react to approval or disapproval

Low:

- Is not bothered by physical discomfort
- Is not attune to emotions on people's faces
- Scratched knee doesn't bother him

7. Persistence -Is the baby's response to certain situations that challenge persistence. A baby who is high in persistence is able to focus their attention and stay with something even when obstacles are put in their path. For example, when learning to walk, a baby who is persistent will fall down many times but will get up again and again regardless of how many times they fall. They will persist until they achieve the standing position and then they will progress quickly onto perfecting walking. Whereas a baby low in persistence will get upset when they fall down, and give up quickly not wanting to persist.

Child

High:

- Continues to practice new skills, whether sports or musical instruments, despite difficulty.

Low:

- Will give up after a few failures, e.g. when starting dance lessons, will quit after the first few lessons if the child feels he/she is not successful
- Gives up on trying to solve a difficult maths problem

8. Distractibility - this is the susceptibility to outside factors distracting the baby from current activity. If a baby is high in distractibility then he is easily redirected from an activity he is doing and easily soothed when he hurts himself. So if we use the above example of when a baby is learning to walk he will fall over many times and hurt himself. A baby who is easily soothed by his mother can be distracted by diverting his attention to a toy or game like 'peek-a-boo' to take his mind off the event that just occurred. A baby who is low in distractibility can be much harder to distract away from the event or feeling of being hurt and will continue to cry.

Child

High:

- Puzzles/homework is always a challenge, as the child is frequently distracted

Low:

- Will focus on completing a construction toy despite many distractions

9. Rhythmicity is the predictability or unpredictability of biological functions. A baby who is high in predictability has an internal body

Chapter Eleven – The Importance of Parenting

clock. They wake at the same time every morning, want their food and will not want to wait until you are ready. They will need their naps at the same time every day. They will have regular and predictable toileting habits. Babies that are low in rhythmicity will wake at different times of the day and night and will have no regular routine. The parent will never be able to predict when they are tired or hungry.

Child

High:

- Creates and follows routines easily
- Is well-organised
- Has predictable behaviour

Low:

- Is disorganised with toys and school work
- Has difficulty being on time
- Finds routines hard to follow

I want to acknowledge that the written information above has been adapted and applied from the 'Roots of Empathy' programme. I currently work as a volunteer instructor on this wonderful programme which teaches school children about empathy through the mother child relationship. Each week I go into the classroom and instruct the children on nine different themes. The children learn by observing the mother and baby who act as the 'teacher' and the children observe from the mother how she responds to her baby's needs. If you would like to know more about the programme, please see the back of this book for the website link.

As a mother it is vitally important to both recognise your baby's temperament but more importantly to work with it rather than against it. You have probably often heard the cliché that you should parent ALL your children the same. In my opinion this could not be further

Chapter Eleven – The Importance of Parenting

from the truth. Every child is unique and will need you as parents to be flexible in your approach to parenting. Let me explain by giving you some case studies using my own four children. I am not going to disclose their names and refer to them all as 'he' to protect their identity.

Baby A

Baby A was a very placid baby; he was high in mood and was always quick to give a smile. He was a curious baby, very mobile and loved to discover new things so we would go to toddler groups, tumble tots and swimming on a weekly basis. Due to being high in activity level he liked being busy and wanted to be on the move constantly. I would have to keep a close eye on him as he was into everything, I couldn't leave him alone for a minute as he was always into things he shouldn't and getting himself into trouble. One day we ended up in A&E as he had managed to put a small object in his ear and I couldn't get it out (yes he was a handful but a lovely handful and lots of fun as well as challenges).

His first reactions to anything new was positive, he loved meeting new people and getting new toys so I would regularly go to the toy library and borrow new toys for him to discover. He was not very high in persistence and would sometimes give up on things easily and get bored quickly, hence my frequent visits to the toy library. He was high in rhythmicity which meant he liked to sleep and eat at regular times so I had to be careful to plan his activities around his sleep and meal times as he got grumpy if he didn't have his sleep or food.

Baby B

Baby B was a very different type of temperament. He was low in mood and cried a lot, it took much more effort to get a smile out of him. I must confess he was the only one of my four babies that I gave a dummy too as I wanted to soothe him from his night crying which was particularly challenging. He was much more cautious as a baby and preferred to be at home. His first reactions were negative, he would cry if a family member went to pick him up and he did not receive cuddles well. He was, however, more persistent than baby A and would stick with things for a long time, especially his crying that could go on for up to an hour (hence the introduction of the dummy- a life saver). He was a very intense baby with a high and demanding cry and wanting his needs met now. He was also quite sensitive and would react badly to any changes and not really adaptable. He was high in all areas of sensitivity both physically (suffering from eczema as a baby) and emotionally. He like, baby A, was high in rhythmicity and wanted to eat and sleep at regular times so again I needed to plan carefully about outside activities, especially with baby B as he would cry loud and hard if he did not get his needs met.

Baby C

Baby C was different again to baby A and B. He was high in mood and loved mischief making. He was always ready with a smile and rarely cried. He was much more adaptable which meant if we were out and about he didn't mind if we were late with lunch or nap time. I could give him some food on the go and he would nap in the car or the pram. He was easy distracted from what he was doing. I tended to put only one or two toys out for him to play with at a time as if he had too many to choose form he would go from one to the other quite quickly and get confused. When feeding him I had to make sure there were not too many distractions as he would get his food all over the place by moving his head. Every sound or object caught his attention –quite tricky and messy. He was high in sensitivity especially about his clothes. He disliked any rough or itchy materials. He hated tags and I would have to cut them all off in order for him to wear them comfortably.

Baby D

Chapter Eleven – The Importance of Parenting

Baby D was different again to my other three children he was the calmest of my four children and never cried but just fussed a little if he wanted feeding or changing. He was a very gentle baby and neither high nor low in mood. He would be happy just to lie in his cot or under the mobile and be content with very little interaction. He was not a demanding baby even when hungry he would be patient and wait. He was also adaptable and would not mind too much about a meal being late or a late nap/bed time. He was low in activity and I could leave him in one position and come back 10-15 minutes later and he would still be in the same position. He was not good with first reactions and did not like meeting new people or going out to activities. He preferred to be at home with me instead. As long as I was close by he was happy.

So you can see from my four children how each was very different and their needs were very different. I had to adapt my parenting to meet their different needs. If I had parented them all the same I would not have been able to meet their different needs. This is so important to be able to adjust your parenting style to meet the needs of each individual baby.

If you reflect back to the chapter on parenting style you may see how different parenting styles could be different to the temperament of your child and cause possible conflict in your child. Of course, your personality may conflict with that of your child and this may cause more challenges and stress for you. It is important to recognise your own personality type, so you can be aware of these challenges that you may face.

To Conclude

They say that parenting comes naturally; this statement in my opinion is one of life's biggest myths. I have seen first-hand how parents struggle in their parenting. You are not alone, for me it was one of the hardest things that I have ever had to learn and master. I am still

Chapter Eleven – The Importance of Parenting

learning after 20yrs of being a parent. You see I had a lot of head knowledge before I had my first baby and assumed I had expert knowledge in the subject of parenting. I thought I knew it ALL when it came to parenting afterall; I had been advising parents on parenting for years before I had my first baby.

Looking back I simply had a lot of 'head knowledge'. I knew what the books said about parenting I had studied them all. However, what I hadn't appreciated as a professional was the need for 'heart knowledge'. I seemed to lose all logic when I became a mother myself and resorted back to being a child in need of nurturing myself.

We, as parents, have in my opinion the hardest and most responsible job in the world. Our job is to grow healthy, happy and successful children. We do our best and will make mistakes along the way. I know as I made many and learned from them. I do know that if you love your children and show them you love them they will forgive your mistakes. This book has been a true and real approach to parenting with a mixture of both personal and professional experience. I hope you have enjoyed reading it and gained new understanding of how our children grow and develop and **how to be your own health visitor** when your baby presents you with challenges as they do and will.

All your baby needs to grow both physically and emotionally is YOU; yes of course they need physical nourishment. They need to have healthy food to grow and achieve their physical milestones. But equally, if not more important, they need love and stimulation to grow emotionally and intellectually to reach their full potential. Feeling safe and loved is so important for children to build their confidence, self-esteem and intellect.

Thank you for reading this book. All that remains is to wish you all **Peaceful Parenting.**

Bibliography

Bates, S. (1979) Practical paediatric Nursing, Blackwell Scientific Publications.

Department of Health (DOH)Birth to five, (2009)Department of Health.

Department of Health Publications, (2009) Reduce the risk of cot death.

Department of Health, The Health Child Programme, Pregnancy and the first five years of life (2009) Department for children, schools and families.

Ding, S and Littleton, K (2005) Children's Personal and Social Development, Blackwell.

Children's Liver Disease Foundation, Jaundice in the newborn baby, Yellow Alert. Caring for young lives, Children's Liver Disease Foundation.

Donaldson, J (2006) Kid's behaviour impacted by lack of sleep, Insight Journal.

Gordon, M ((2005) Roots of Empathy-Changing the World Child By Child, Thomas Allen.

Health Promotion Public Health (2013).Postnatal Depression.

Millpond (2005)Teach your child to sleep, Hamlyns.

My Personal Health Held Record (Red Book), NHS.

National Screening Committee (2011). Screening tests for baby.

Oates, J. Wood, C and Grayson, A. (2005) Psychological Development and Early Childhood, Blackwell.

Sheridan, M,D. (1975) From Birth to Five Years Children's Developmental Progress, Routledge.

Unicef UK Baby Freindly Initative, (2010). The health professional's guide to:"A guide to infant formula for parents who are bottle feeding", Unicef UK.

Unicef UK Baby Friendly Initiative (2008). Three –day course in Breastfeeding management-Participant's handbook. Unicef UK.

www.nhs.uk/Conditions/Postnataldepression/Pages/Diagnosis.aspx

About the Author

Ann Guindi has worked with children for the past thirty years both in health and education. She started out as a Sick Children's Nurse and worked for 8 years in the acute sector. Her area of expertise was cardiothoracic medical and surgical care of babies and children in need of heart/lung transplants and corrective lifesaving surgery at Great Ormond Street Hospital.

In 1990 she retrained as a Health Visitor (HV) and moved into the community as she wanted to do more preventative work. She has been a HV for 20, years working primarily in South East London. Her main role was in health education and promotion, working with young families and the under 5's.

In 2003 she moved from the health service into education and set up her own family business, Happy Faces Montessori Ltd, a preschool and Baby Unit in SE London. She sold both nurseries in 2008 to spend more time with her family.

Since then Ann has been self-employed working as an early years consultant, lecturer, assessor, coach, mentor and inspector for various organisations.

These include Greenwich University where she lectured in Early Years in Leadership and Management and also acted as a mentor and assessor to the students on the various pathways during their studies to gain Early Years professional Status (EYPs). Ann herself has undergone this training and holds this status.

Ann has been an assessor for the Montessori Evaluation and accreditation Board (MEAB) assessing preschools to see if they are adhering to the Montessori philosophy and teaching methods. She has also been a lead inspector for the Independent Schools Inspectorate (ISI) ensuring that Schools are maintaining the welfare and safety of children along with delivering the Early Years Foundation Stage Curriculum (EYFS).

Since 2010 Ann has been running a personal development business **'Hope Dream Believe'** her niche areas are working with parents and other businesses. She loves helping others achieve their personal and business goals in life. Please visit www.hopedreambelieve.co.uk. Her special interests include Neuro Linguistic Programming, personality profiling and coaching.

Ann believes in giving back to the community and has carried out a number of voluntary roles in her capacity as a counsellor, including working at Greenwich University (student counsellor), Bromley Y (a youth organisation), Queen Marys Hospital (counselling terminally ill cancer patients) and the P2b - place to be (school counsellor/play therapist).

Ann is currently working as a volunteer with the 'Roots of Empathy' teaching children about empathy through a 'baby teacher' as it is a proven method of reducing aggression and bullying in schools. www.rootsofempathy.org

Ann's other interests are the promotion of pro-social behaviour in children and working with victims of domestic violence as a 'Freedom Programme' facilitator.

Ann is also a protégé student with the Coaching Academy and working towards her diploma in youth Impact Coaching.

Ann is using all her knowledge, skills and experience gained over the last 30 years in working with children and parents to launch her new business **'Parenting Peace'** as she believes you, the parent want to do the best for your children and she believes she can help you in that very important role. Please see www.parentingpeace.co.uk for more information.

Ann is married to Chris and they have four children, Ben, Joe, Ollie and Sophie.

Qualifications:

Registered Sick Children's' Nurse (1985)

Registered General Nurse (1988)

Registered Health Visitor (1991)

Montessori Teaching Diploma (1996)

BSc (Hons) Professional Practice (Nursing) (1999)

Early Years Professional Status (2007)

NLP Practitioner, Time line Therapy, Hypnotherapy and Coaching (2009)

MSc Therapeutic Counselling (2010)

Master Practitioner NLP/Life Coach (2010)

NLP Master Practitioner, Time line Therapy, Hypnotherapy and Coaching (2010)

Life Performance Coach (2010)

BSc (Hons) Psychology (2011)

CPD Diploma Coaching (2011)

Personality D.I.S.C Profiler and Myers Briggs Trainer (2011)

CMI level 5 Leadership and Management (2012)

Prince 2 Foundation and Practitioner (2013)

Business Coaching Diploma (2014)

Freedom Programme Facilitator (2014)

Index

A

abuse · 17, 65, 219
Ages and Stages Questionnaire' · 27
allergy · 104, 105, 106, 127
antenatal · 8, 13, 14, 33, 84, 145
antenatal assessment · 8
Anxiety · 13, 158, 162
asthma · 9
attachment · 221, 222
Au-pair · 152
Authoritarian · 14, 219

B

baby · 3, 1, 4, 5, 6, 8, 9, 12, 14, 15, 17, 18, 19, 20, 21, 22, 23, 25, 27, 31, 32, 33, 34, 35, 37, 39, 40, 41, 42, 43, 44, 45, 46, 47, 48, 49, 50, 52, 53, 54, 57, 59, 60, 61, 64, 65, 66, 68, 69, 70, 71, 72, 73, 74, 75, 76, 78, 79, 80, 81, 82, 83, 84, 85, 95, 98, 99, 100, 101, 102, 105, 106, 108, 109, 110, 112, 113, 114, 116, 117, 118, 120, 121, 122, 123, 124, 125, 126, 127, 128, 129, 130, 131, 132, 133, 134, 135, 136, 137, 140, 141, 142, 143, 144, 145, 146, 147, 148, 149, 150, 151, 152, 153, 155, 156, 157, 159, 160, 161, 163, 166, 171, 172, 173, 174, 179, 180, 181, 182, 183, 184, 185, 186, 187, 188, 194, 195, 199, 202, 203, 204, 205, 206, 207, 208, 209, 210, 216, 222, 223, 225, 226, 227, 228, 229, 230, 231, 232, 233, 234, 235, 236, 237, 238, 241
bacteria · 52, 57, 58, 74, 149
BCG · 8, 24, 51, 52, 141
behaviour · 71, 157, 159, 163, 166, 169, 170, 172, 173, 174, 175, 177, 178, 192, 200, 201, 210, 216, 218, 219, 221, 223, 232, 238
birth · 7, 4, 9, 12, 13, 14, 15, 17, 19, 20, 21, 22, 23, 24, 25, 29, 32, 33, 34, 35, 36, 37, 39, 40, 41, 46, 64, 65, 66, 68, 70, 74, 75, 80, 83, 84, 85, 100, 108, 113, 115, 116, 117, 118, 120, 122, 125, 140, 141, 145, 150, 179, 180, 201, 202, 216
birth certificate · 64, 65, 66
bones · 33, 39, 52, 99, 147, 151
booster · 55
bottle · 14, 15, 37, 41, 60, 73, 96, 99, 101, 108, 109, 110, 112, 122, 126, 128, 129, 132, 134, 135, 138, 150, 151, 158, 160, 172, 182, 239
bottle feeding · 15, 122, 129, 239
breast milk · 40, 69, 71, 78, 79, 82, 97, 98, 101, 103, 106, 126, 146
breastfeeding · 15, 19, 40, 42, 44, 45, 69, 71, 72, 74, 75, 79, 81, 82, 126, 137, 141
Breasts · 24
breathing · 15, 43, 56, 74, 100, 107, 138, 144
breech · 143

C

c- section · 33
casein dominant · 98, 99
cervix · 82, 83

Index

Childcare · 11, 151, 153
Childminder · 152
choking · 56, 97, 108, 149
circumcision · 47
classes · 13, 14, 15, 18, 19, 155
clinic · 5, 17, 24, 25, 29, 31, 52, 54, 56, 82, 83, 93, 114, 117, 125, 140, 141, 144, 145, 150, 165
colic · 105, 107, 113, 114, 132, 133
Communication · 13, 27, 183, 184, 206, 210
Community Staff Nurses · 6
complications · 14, 37, 47, 58, 78
condensed milks · 102
coning · 39
conjunctivitis · 40
constipated · 121, 134, 135
contraception · 81, 82
Contraception · 24
Controlled crying · 163
cot death · 12, 24, 48, 49, 238
cow's milk · 96, 102, 103
CSN · 6, 27
culture · 117, 155, 215, 216
Cystic Fibrosis · 21

D

dehydrated · 39, 71, 130, 151
delivery · 6, 14, 37, 39, 68, 80, 126
delivery suite · 14
Democratic parenting · 220
depressed · 9, 24, 84, 173
depression · 13, 16, 18, 19, 24, 83, 84, 93, 94, 140, 142, 158
development · 5, 6, 7, 27, 29, 31, 32, 148, 159, 179, 180, 183, 190, 196, 201, 202, 203, 204, 205, 214, 216, 218, 219, 241
diabetes · 9, 13

diarrhoea · 51, 82, 103, 118, 130, 137, 138, 139
diet · 13, 101, 103, 137, 148
Diphtheria · 8, 54, 55, 56
discharge · 20, 22, 34, 40, 107
discipline · 214
disease · 51, 52, 56, 62, 82, 102, 105, 107
distractibility · 231
domestic violence · 12
Domestic Violence · 14
drinking · 12, 13, 39, 50, 62, 142
drug-taking · 12, 13

E

eczema · 9, 105, 234
Edinburgh Post Natal Depression Score · 84
education · 3, 5, 6, 18, 146, 240
emotions · 3, 4, 165, 180, 229, 230
EPDS · 9, 84, 85, 86, 93
ethnicity · 125
evaporated milk · 102
Exercise · 13
experience · 3, 1, 2, 4, 12, 14, 15, 18, 22, 24, 37, 39, 68, 74, 85, 129, 133, 141, 145, 155, 167, 180, 193, 197, 202, 214, 215, 237, 241
eyes · 38, 40, 41, 46, 106, 108, 130, 142, 181, 189, 195, 228

F

family support worker · 11
family tree · 9
Feeding · 1, 9, 25, 79, 95, 141
fetal conditions · 7
fever · 53, 60

Index

financial · 16, 65
Fine motor · 27, 183
Follow up · 11, 83, 140, 141
Follow-on formula · 101
fontanelle · 26, 39, 138
formula · 79, 95, 96, 97, 98, 99, 101, 103, 104, 105, 106, 108, 122, 126, 129, 132, 133, 135, 137, 146, 151, 239
frenulum · 44

G

gastroenteritis · 51, 138
genes · 204
Genitals · 26
genogram · 9
goat's milk · 102, 103
GP · 9, 6, 17, 26, 32, 34, 40, 42, 45, 48, 52, 53, 54, 56, 60, 61, 62, 64, 65, 66, 80, 82, 84, 89, 93, 104, 108, 118, 126, 127, 129, 130, 131, 134, 141, 142, 143, 144, 184, 194
Gross motor · 27, 183
guidelines · 7, 97

H

Haemophilus influenza · 54, 55, 57
HCP · 6, 7, 25
head · 6, 33, 38, 39, 50, 61
health · 3, 5, 1, 3, 4, 5, 6, 7, 8, 9, 12, 13, 15, 16, 17, 18, 20, 22, 23, 24, 27, 29, 30, 31, 32, 35, 48, 56, 60, 69, 75, 82, 83, 93, 96, 112, 114, 118, 123, 142, 143, 146, 158, 169, 179, 183, 190, 216, 237, 239, 240
health visitor · 3, 5, 1, 3, 4, 15, 18, 35, 69, 75, 114, 169, 216, 237

Health Visitor Implementation Plan · 1
Healthy Child Programme · 16, 25
hearing · 20, 21, 180, 181
heart · 26, 33, 56, 74, 138, 143, 144, 145, 165, 237, 240
heartbeat · 19
hips · 33, 143, 184
history · 12, 65, 102, 105, 202
home inspection · 8
home visits · 5, 7
hospital · 3, 4, 14, 19, 20, 21, 22, 33, 34, 35, 41, 44, 45, 62, 64, 66, 80, 131, 142, 145
Housing · 14
hunger · 95, 113, 159
Hypothyroidism · 21

I

imitation games · 210
immune system · 159
immunisations · 54, 56, 59
Immunisations · 7, 8, 25, 51
Income · 14
infection · 37, 42, 44, 48, 52, 57, 58, 69, 73, 118, 131, 137
injection · 20, 37, 51, 53, 61
interaction · 13, 214, 235
intercourse · 80, 81, 215, 216
irritability · 131, 138

J

jaundice · 22, 37, 40, 41, 42
Jaundice · 40, 41
juice · 97, 134, 135, 136, 139

Index

L

labour · 14, 15, 18, 19, 68, 74, 216
language · 27, 155, 173, 180, 202, 206
lifestyle · 12
lungs · 26, 33, 52, 132

M

mastitis · 69, 71, 73, 76
Mastitis · 73
Maternal · 9, 12, 64, 140
maternal health · 1
measles · 58, 59, 62, 63
Measles · 8, 55, 58, 63
medication · 44, 93, 129, 145
Men C · 54, 55
midwife · 7, 8, 19, 21, 22, 34, 35, 41, 42, 68, 69, 93
milk · 10, 40, 43, 68, 69, 70, 71, 73, 74, 76, 79, 95, 96, 97, 98, 99, 101, 102, 103, 104, 105, 106, 108, 109, 110, 112, 113, 116, 120, 122, 123, 124, 126, 127, 129, 131, 133, 136, 146, 147, 150, 151
minerals · 96, 103
mistakes · 2, 3, 220, 237
MMR · 8, 55, 58, 62
mood · 25, 93, 140, 142, 227, 233, 234, 235
mother · 5, 2, 4, 11, 15, 16, 18, 22, 23, 24, 25, 35, 37, 44, 64, 65, 69, 76, 79, 81, 83, 84, 93, 96, 99, 100, 141, 145, 146, 151, 165, 171, 172, 177, 200, 210, 214, 216, 221, 222, 223, 225, 227, 228, 231, 233, 237
mouth · 33, 43, 44, 61, 72, 79, 95, 107, 108, 109, 112, 114, 130, 146, 148, 149, 174, 181, 182, 186, 187, 195, 201
Mumps · 8, 55, 58, 59, 63
muscle cramps · 100
myths · 3, 236

N

nanny · 152, 153
nap · 160, 226, 229, 235
nappy · 34, 46, 47, 95, 137, 172, 173, 208, 230
National Childbirth Trust · 15
National Institute for Clinical Excellence · 83
NCT · 15, 18, 19
neglect · 17
nervous system · 56, 57
Neuroscience · 13, 199, 203
new parents · 1, 95, 149
newborn · 20, 21, 41, 99, 129, 133, 142, 143, 145, 180, 238
NICE · 7, 83
Night Terrors · 12, 167
nightmare · 167, 168, 193
nipples · 44, 69, 71, 72, 73
NN · 6, 27
nose · 40, 43, 78, 95, 107, 189, 195
nourishment · 103, 146, 237
nursery · 6, 18, 29, 139, 151, 152, 153, 155, 156, 172, 192, 194, 196, 211, 228
nursery nurses · 6, 18
Nutrition · 13, 104
nutritional content · 96

O

oestrogen · 81, 82

Index

ointment · 47
ovaries · 59

P

Paediatric Dietician · 104
panic attacks · 13
parenting · 3, 1, 3, 5, 120, 140, 171, 178, 193, 215, 216, 218, 219, 220, 221, 222, 233, 236, 237
parents · 3, 4, 7, 8, 9, 15, 16, 20, 27, 31, 32, 39, 46, 49, 62, 63, 65, 80
Permissive parenting · 219
personality · 192, 216, 218, 224, 225, 236
Pertussis · 8, 54, 55, 56
Phenylketonuria · 21
Pneumococcal · 8, 54, 55, 57, 58
Polio · 8, 54, 55, 57
positive parenting · 221
possetting · 123
post-natal · 24
pre term · 108
pregnancy · 7, 11, 12, 33, 35, 37, 49, 57, 59, 80, 81, 84, 216
premature · 34, 37, 42
preschool · 55, 240
prevention · 3, 32, 48, 49, 137, 173
Problem Solving · 13, 14, 27, 183, 186, 191, 208, 212
problems · 14, 16, 22, 32, 34, 37, 45, 56, 61, 73, 76, 98, 113, 123, 125, 133, 142, 143, 157, 158, 159, 161, 203
protein · 101, 103, 129, 133
psychological development · 199
psychological health · 83
psychologist · 93, 175, 199, 200, 222
Public Health Nurse · 4
pyloric stenosis · 127

Q

questionnaire · 27
questions · 11, 27, 31, 84, 92, 112, 114, 120, 142, 195, 196, 197, 213, 215

R

rash · 44, 46, 47, 58, 59, 62
red book · 23, 35, 36, 65, 116, 125, 141
reflex · 33, 123, 127, 149, 184
reflux · 105, 107, 129
registration · 64, 65
rehydration solutions · 131, 137, 138
rickets · 99
risk · 7, 9, 11, 12, 15, 17, 19, 51, 57, 65, 82, 96, 104, 108, 130, 132, 137, 149, 150, 238
Rubella · 8, 55, 58, 59, 63

S

school · 4, 17, 18, 29, 35, 58, 65, 83, 152, 155, 167, 197, 215, 232, 233, 241
screening · 5, 7, 14, 20, 21, 25, 27, 33, 82, 84, 145, 179
secure attachment · 222
sensory stimulation · 203, 230
Sexual Health · 13
sheep's milk · 102, 103
Sibling Rivalry · 12, 171
sick · 3, 1, 3, 4, 5, 6, 34, 106, 113, 121, 124, 152, 153, 163
Sickle cell anaemia · 21
SIDS · 7, 12, 49

Index

single mothers · 9
skill mix · 6, 17, 27
skill mix team · 6, 27
skills · 3, 1, 4, 6, 204, 212, 214, 218, 231, 241
skin · 33, 40, 41, 44, 46, 47, 50, 53, 61, 62, 68, 70, 73, 74, 75, 76, 105, 106, 130, 138, 180, 184
sleep · 19, 49, 50, 80, 95, 131, 142, 157, 158, 159, 160, 161, 162, 163, 165, 167, 168, 169, 171, 181, 200, 226, 228, 234, 238
sleep training · 157
Sleeping · 1, 25
smoking · 12
Smoking · 13
social services · 11
social worker · 17
solid food · 106, 132, 146, 151, 159
Soya · 10, 103, 104, 108
Spina Bifida · 33
spontaneous vaginal delivery · 37
sterilisation · 15
stools · 41, 42, 47, 105, 107, 120, 126, 133, 135, 137, 139
support · 1, 3, 4, 5, 9, 11, 15, 16, 17, 22, 24, 25, 28, 29, 67, 69, 72, 75, 79, 84, 85, 89, 94, 98, 99, 117, 144, 146, 156, 185, 216
surgery · 26, 54, 56, 65, 141, 145, 240
swelling · 59, 61, 62, 107

T

tantrums · 169, 171, 175, 192
TB · 8, 51, 52
teat · 97, 108, 109, 110, 112, 128, 132
teeth · 99, 100, 146, 147, 150, 151
temperament · 224, 233, 234, 236
temperature · 34, 49, 53, 58, 59, 61, 62, 74, 126, 131, 136, 161, 203, 230
testicles · 34, 59, 144, 184
Tetanus · 8, 54, 55, 56
Thallasceamia · 21
toilet training · 193
tongue · 43, 44, 105, 106, 108, 109, 146, 148, 180, 182
Tonsillitis · 131
training · 3, 5, 6, 136, 159, 172, 193, 194, 200, 218, 240
Tuberculosis · 51
twin · 11

U

urine · 41, 42, 68, 81, 138, 194

V

vaccine · 51, 52, 57, 58, 62, 63
Vitamin D · 9, 24, 99, 100, 101
vitamins · 33, 96
vocabulary · 189, 195, 196, 197
vomiting · 51, 82, 98, 107, 110, 123, 124, 127, 130, 135, 138, 139

W

walking · 100, 188, 190, 231
Weaning · 1, 11, 140, 146
weight · 14, 22, 26, 27, 31, 34, 70, 99, 106, 107, 108, 113, 116, 118, 120, 121, 122, 125, 129, 135, 139, 141, 144, 145, 148, 149, 190, 202
Weight loss · 53
whey dominant · 98, 99
whooping cough · 54, 55, 57

Index

Whooping cough · 56
wind · 110, 112, 127, 128, 132
work · 5, 1, 3, 4, 6, 8, 9, 12, 23, 38, 60, 69, 79, 93, 94, 112, 129, 133, 134, 141, 145, 151, 155, 156, 158, 159, 165, 175, 193, 195, 206, 212, 214, 228, 232, 233, 240

Printed in Great Britain
by Amazon.co.uk, Ltd.,
Marston Gate.